Make Your Hand Sanitizer

A Step-By-Step Guide to Make Your Own 99 Natural Homemade Hand Wipes, Spray, Sanitizer, and Liquid Soap to Kill Germs, Viruses, and Bacteria For a Healthier Lifestyle

Veronica Martel

Table of Contents

Hydrogen Peroxide Sanitizer

Aloe Vera Gel Sanitizer

Lemon Sanitizer

Lavender and Tea Tree Oil Sanitizer

Orange Sanitizer

Eucalyptus Oil Sanitizer

Green Apple Sanitizer

Grapefruit Sanitizer

Tea Tree and Eucalyptus Oil Sanitizer

Peppermint Oil Sanitizer

Orange and Tea Tree Oil Sanitizer

Lavender Sanitizer

Orange and Cinnamon Sanitizer

Lime Oil Sanitizer

Vitamin E and Sweet Orange Sanitizer

Cinnamon And Lemongrass Oil Sanitizer

Cardamom Sanitizer

Chamomile Sanitizer

Rose Sanitizer

Jasmine Sanitizer

Caraway Sanitizer

Fennel Sanitizer

Lychee Sanitizer

Anise Oil Sanitizer

Balsam Fir Oil Sanitizer

Ylang Ylang Sanitizer

Lemongrass Sanitizer

Frankincense Sanitizer

Vanilla Sanitizer

Calamus Oil Sanitizer

Calamondin Oil Sanitizer

Davana Oil Sanitizer

Patchouli Sanitizer

Galbanum Oil Sanitizer

May Chang Oil Sanitizer

Cedarwood Sanitizer

Cypress Sanitizer

Palmarosa Oil Sanitizer

Three-Oils Sanitizer

Hyssop Sanitizer

Vetiver Oil Sanitizer

Strawberry Sanitizer

Lavender and Vitamin E Sanitizer

Four-Oils Sanitizer

Oregano Sanitizer

Four-Oils and Glycerin Sanitizer

Juniper Sanitizer

Turmeric Sanitizer

Cinnamon Sanitizer

Lemon Balm Sanitizer

Myrrha Sanitizer

Clove Sanitizer

Rosemary Sanitizer

Citronella Sanitizer

Sage Sanitizer

Tea Tree Sanitizer

Sandalwood Sanitizer

Ginger Oil Sanitizer

Tarragon Oil Sanitizer

Thyme Oil Sanitizer

Pine Oil Sanitizer

Tsuga Oil Sanitizer

Star Anise Sanitizer

Rosewood Sanitizer

Emil Oil Sanitizer

Agar Oil Sanitizer

Fenugreek Sanitizer

Balsam of Peru Sanitizer

Basil Sanitizer

Bergamot Sanitizer

Black Pepper Oil Sanitizer

Citronella Sanitizer

Cidron Oil Sanitizer

Salvia Sclarea Oil Sanitizer

Melissa Oil Sanitizer

Moringa Sanitizer

Thyme Oil and Vitamin E Sanitizer

Rose Mary and Lemongrass Sanitizer

Conclusion

Introduction

Congratulations on purchasing *Make Your Own Hand Sanitizer: A Step-By-Step Guide To Make Your Own Natural Homemade Hand Wipes, Spray, Sanitizer, and Liquid Soap to Kill Germs, Viruses and Bacteria For a Healthier Lifestyle* and thank you for doing so.

At this time, when the whole world is buying sanitizers to the point that it is no longer available in certain markets, it is now of utmost importance that you learn to make your own sanitizers. In this way, you will not have to depend on anyone and yet maintain your personal hygiene. The importance of hygiene in our lives cannot be expressed in words and is indispensable. You are shaking hands with people, holding doors open, and also touching other public places and then you are holding food items with that same hand. This is how germs are spread and diseases are caused. But all of that can be stopped if you start using sanitizers.

In this book, I am going to show you how easy it is to make your own hand sanitizer at home with some simple ingredients. I am also going to give you a brief introduction of what hygiene is and how important it is to mankind.

There are plenty of books on this subject on the market, thanks again for choosing this one! Every effort was made to ensure it is full of as much useful information as possible; please enjoy it!

Medical Disclaimer: Every detail mentioned in this book is for the purpose of information only and you should not replace it with a doctor's advice. All information in this book has been provided in good faith but I do not promise a warranty of any kind nor do I imply or express adequacy, accuracy, or completeness of the information present here.

Chapter 1: Importance of Hygiene

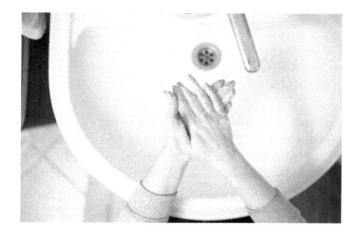

Have you ever thought why you wake up early, brush and get washed up? Is it just because you were taught to do so from a young age? No. It is a lot more than just a routine that you follow. You are just practicing good personal hygiene. Hygiene is an ornamental word that we often use to refer to clean habits to follow a healthy lifestyle. There are a lot of reasons why we need to clean ourselves regularly. These include removing dirt from our body, food particles from our teeth, getting rid of germs, and bodily secretions. It is a fundamental part of our life to maintain proper hygiene techniques. In this chapter, I will try to exhibit some of the compelling steps that you need to follow to stay hygienic. But before that, we will take a glance at what hygiene means to understand this topic better.

What is Hygiene?

Hygiene is a set of usual procedures that we follow to preserve our health. It is our regular duty to clean our bodies so that we are less prone to diseases and are capable of preventing the transmission of unwanted particles. Maintaining cleanliness and performing regular duties goes hand in hand.

Many people confuse hygiene with being clean, which is not the matter. Hygiene is rather a broader aspect. It is completely dependent on the personal choices that an individual makes, which depends on the frequency of taking a shower, washing hands and clothes, trimming fingernails. It even includes paying attention to keeping our home and workplace, specifically bathroom facilities, fresh and dirt-free. It is all about maintaining proper self-esteem to make your-self look and feel better, which keeps you motivated and brings out the best in you every day. It is always our foremost role to perform these duties that will help us to rise and shine and lead a healthy life.

A Step-by-Step Personal Hygiene Routine to Follow

1. **Bathing** – It is important to wash your hair and body at regular intervals, if not regularly. Basically, you need to follow the routine that works for you, keeping in mind that it will ultimately do you good by enhancing your overall health. Showering with warm water and soap every day helps to keep germs away and keep your body dirt-free. You can even consider bathing twice a day when the weather is moderately hot. Bathing plays an

integral role in maintaining good health in the following ways:

- Bathing with soap and water helps to kill bacteria which causes odor.
- Infections like Athlete's Foot can be checked upon by cleaning and drying infected areas daily.
- Shampoo and conditioning the hair helps to keep the scalp clean and free from head lice.

2. **Hand Washing** – Washing your hands is the primary step towards being clean and hygienic because these are the two organs we are using constantly from waking up in the morning to going back to bed. We can sense that our hands are the biggest shipper of pathogens. We are constantly touching different areas, using our cell-phone, shaking our hands with people. Therefore it is very important to keep them clean. Maintaining hand hygiene is the easiest and quickest way of ensuring that our family and people we work with are safe. Illnesses such as cold, cough, flu, which are easily spread, can be stopped by washing your hands. Washing your hands prior to eating and after you are completed, before preparing food, sneezing or coughing, after using the washroom and even after managing the garbage can guide you to a better disease-free life.

3. **Brushing and Flossing** – Teeth deserve maximum priority. Besides playing an apparent role in eating, they would grind the

food into smaller pieces helping to swallow the particles. Teeth are considered as the climactic glory of your body and hence make you attractive, push up your confidence, and give you the tag of sociable. Therefore it is necessary to keep them healthy for sustenance, better interaction, and social allure and to avoid crucial problems in the future. Oral hygiene needs to be practiced to avoid tooth decay, gum problems, and several infections. All you are required to do is brush your teeth twice a day, floss them regularly, store the brush in a dry and clean place, and visit the dentist at an interval of six months to carry a healthy smile wherever you go.

4. **Trimming Your Nails** – Trim your toe and fingernails to prevent problems such as infected nail beds and hangnails. Do not forget to keep them in good shape.

5. **Sleeping Tight** – Getting a good sleep of about ten hours is priceless. Sleeping is the time when our body gets proper rest, which helps to boost up our immune system. A night of good sleep is irreplaceable and helps you to feel refreshed and do out daily household chores. If you are unwilling to put the natural defenses of your body to jeopardy, do get a good sleep.

What Happens When You Have Poor Hygiene?

Managing a proper hygiene routine is an essential part of living. It is directly akin to lower ailment and better health. Poor hygienic habits can lead to minor aftereffect, which ultimately makes way to serious health issues.

Not washing hands can bring about the transfer of germs to mouth and eyes and can cause other issues like stomach viruses. Not taking good care of the teeth can cause serious issues like the formation of plaque and other health issues like heart disease. There are several other diseases caused due to poor personal hygiene which include scabies, head lice, ringworm, body lice, swimmer's ear, diarrhea, pinworms, pubic lice, hot tub rash, etc. These diseases can be prevented by following proper hygiene habits.

A positive attitude can be maintained by following the hygiene habits regularly. This can help you to look presentable, make you feel good and worthy, make you believe in yourself, and, most importantly, gift you with a strong and vigorous lifestyle.

Chapter 2: Homemade Sanitizers and Their Importance

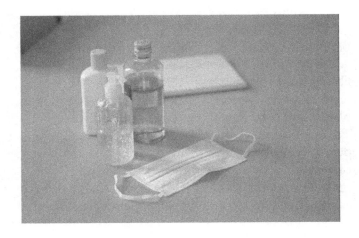

First introduced in medical settings in the year 1966, hand sanitizers became popular in the early 1990s. Available as liquids, foams or gels, they are generally used to decrease the presence of infectious agents on the hands. In healthcare settings, alcohol-based formulations are preferred to washing hands with soap and water. Alcohol, as an antiseptic, has been used as early as 1963.

Hand sanitizers are an effective and convenient way of cleaning your hands when soap and water are unavailable. Alcohol-based hand sanitizers contain several combinations of isopropyl alcohol, ethyl alcohol or propanol. The most effective versions of sanitizers contain about 60% to 90% alcohol. They can kill a wide variety of microorganisms, but they cannot kill spores. Non-alcoholic versions of hand sanitizers are also available. They generally contain triclosan or benzalkonium chloride.

How Do Hand Sanitizers Work?

Alcohol is the main ingredient in most hand sanitizers. Alcohols are organic molecules composed of hydrogen, oxygen, and carbon. Ethanol, propanol, and isopropyl alcohol are common chemicals that are used in disinfectants as they are highly soluble in water.

According to a review published in the journal 'Clinical Microbiology Reviews' in 2014, alcohol can kill disease-causing microorganisms and pathogens by splitting up proteins, breaking cells into pieces, or destroying the metabolism of the cell. Solutions having as little as 30% alcohol can kill certain pathogens. Their effectiveness increases with an increase in the concentration of alcohol.

According to studies, solutions having a concentration of more than 60% alcohol can kill a wider variety of bacteria and viruses. As the concentration of alcohol increases, they work faster. However, the solutions having a concentration of about 90 to 95% alcohol seem to be most effective in killing microorganisms. Moreover, alcohol doesn't lose its effectiveness with continued use because the microorganisms that it kills cannot develop any resistance to it.

According to a review made in 2014, ethanol is so powerful that in high concentrations, it can kill 3 species of disease cause bacteria – *E. coli*, *Staphylococcus saprophyticus*, and *Serratia marcescens* which cannot be killed by washing hands with soap and water. Alcohol, however, cannot kill germs like norovirus, *Cryptosporidium*, or *Clostridium difficile*.

A few small-scale pieces of research show that alcohol-free hand sanitizers having benzalkonium chloride as the main ingredient at a concentration of 0.13 percent, are just as effective at getting rid of harmful microorganisms. However, there isn't any independent research that shows that it's better than alcohol-containing hand sanitizers. According to the Centre for Disease Control and Prevention, alcohol-free hand sanitizers only reduce the growth of germs rather than killing them. It is recommended by the CDC that hand sanitizers should have at least 60% alcohol in them for maximum effectiveness.

Purpose of Sanitizers

Even though your hands serve a lot of important purposes, they also put your eyes, mouth, nose, and several other parts of your body in contact with germs and make you sick. That's why it's important to keep your hands clean. Washing your hands with warm water and soap several times a day is the best way to clean them, but cleaning them with hand sanitizers is also a worthy alternative.

To use a hand sanitizer you just have to apply enough of the product on your hands so that it can cover all surfaces and then rub your hands together for about twenty seconds until they feel dry. You should not rinse or wipe your hands before the sanitizer has dried. Always use a sanitizer that has at least 60 percent alcohol content. At home, schools and childcare facilities, children should use hand sanitizers under adult supervision to prevent them from swallowing it.

Always use a hand sanitizer that contains alcohol before and after visiting a loved one in a nursing home or hospital. However, if the person is sick with *Clostridium difficile*, be sure to wash your hands with soap and water.

The workplace is a hotbed for bacteria and germs. Starting from Monday to Friday, Americans spend more time in their workplace than anywhere else. Throughout the day, employees have to write up reports, open doors, greet new clients and perform many such activities using their hands. All these activities end up exposing them to harmful bacteria and germs. It is very important to implement a proper hand hygiene program at the workplace, considering that about 80% of all infectious diseases are transmitted by hands. Moreover, almost 90% of office workers go to work even if they are sick because of the ever-growing workload. According to the CDC, the flu costs businesses about 10.4 billion dollars every year for outpatient visits and hospitalizations. To reduce absenteeism and associated costs by more than 40%, proper hand hygiene compliance is necessary. As washing hands with soap and water isn't always a viable option; keeping hand sanitizers in strategic places throughout the office is one of the best ways to avoid getting sick and spreading diseases. Keeping hand sanitizers in high traffic areas could also encourage the employees to maintain a healthier working environment in the office by improving their hand hygiene.

Benefits of Hand Sanitizers

1. **Cleanliness** – One of the most important benefits of hand sanitizers is that they kill germs. Hand sanitizers can kill 99.9% of the germs present on your hands if you use it correctly. It is recommended by the CDC that you wash your hands every time you are around animals, food, garbage, etc. Hand sanitizers are a perfect addition to using soap and water to wash your hands.

2. **Portability** – In some situations, when you need to wash your hands and soap and water are not available, you can easily use hand sanitizers. You can always keep a small bottle of hand sanitizer with you in your purse, glove compartment or even in your pocket.

3. **Less risk of disease** – Minimizing your exposure to other people's germs during the flu season is very important for your health. You can reduce your chances of getting sick by sanitizing your hands a few times throughout the day.

4. **Great for group settings** – Germs can spread quickly in places that have lots of foot traffic like classrooms and offices. In close quarters, other people's germs can easily affect you. That is why keeping a hand sanitizer is ideal in group settings.

Limitations of Hand Sanitizers

Although hand sanitizers can be very useful when soap and water are unavailable, they have a few drawbacks. Some of the limitations of hand sanitizers are:

- All hand sanitizers are not created equally. Check the active ingredients present in the sanitizer. The acceptable forms of alcohol are ethanol, isopropanol or propanol. However, be certain that the concentration of alcohol in the bottle is between 60% and 90%. Alcohol content below 60% is not enough to be effective.

- Alcohol-based hand sanitizers can quickly eliminate a wide variety of microbes from your hands but they cannot eliminate all kinds of germs. For eliminating certain kinds of germs, like norovirus, *Cryptosporidium*, and *Clostridium difficile*, soap and water is more effective than alcohol-based hand sanitizers.

- Although alcohol-based hand sanitizers can effectively destroy a variety of microbes when they are correctly used, many people might not use a volume that's large enough to kill the germs or they might wipe off the sanitizer before it has dried.

- If your hands are visibly dirty or greasy, hand sanitizers might not be as effective. Various studies show that hand sanitizers work effectively in medical settings such as hospitals, where your hands come in contact with germs but don't get heavily soiled or greasy. Some researchers also show that hand sanitizers might work effectively against certain kinds of germs on slightly soiled hands.

- However, in community settings, like when you play sports, handle food, go camping or fishing, or while working in the garden, your hands might become very soiled and greasy. In such situations, when your hands get very greasy or soiled, hand sanitizers may not work well. It is recommended to wash hands with soap and water in such situations.

- Hand sanitizers might not be able to eliminate harmful chemicals such as pesticides and heavy metals from your hands. A few studies show that hand sanitizers cannot eliminate or inactivate several types of harmful chemicals. If your hands have come in contact with harmful chemicals, wash properly with soap and water.

- Hand sanitizers containing ethyl alcohol or ethanol are safe if you use them as directed. However, if a person swallows more than a few mouthfuls of sanitizers, it can cause alcohol poisoning. Hand sanitizers should be kept out of reach of children and should not be used without adult supervision as children may be tempted to swallow sanitizers that are brightly colored, scented and attractively packed.

Making the use of hand sanitizers a habit can decrease your chances of illness by keeping you exposed to fewer germs. Take some time to rub some sanitizer on your hands irrespective of whether you are on a playground or a hospital. It's an easy step to being healthier.

Chapter 3: Things to Know Before Making Your Own Hand Sanitizer

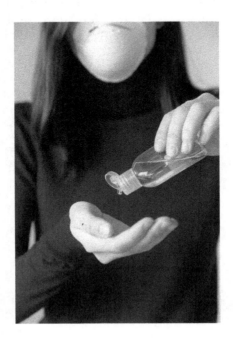

It was not until the outbreak of this deadly virus named Corona (official name – COVID -19) that the idea of making our sanitizer became so popular. This virus has caused a lot of panics all over the world leading to the sell-out of basic amenities like water, foods which are not perishable, toilet paper at an incredibly fast rate. Another hot product that is disappearing at an even faster rate is nothing but the hand sanitizer. Our store shelves are finding it hard to provide us with hand sanitizers as thousands are rushing to stockpile the supplies. Even the online retailing companies are facing a hard time with keeping this product in their stock because of its increased demand.

Since we are running short of this important amenity, the very next thing that we are making our mind think about is preparing one for ourselves and our family members. And if you think that it is just about alcohol, let me correct you and provide you with advice, that it is a more complicated thing. As per the insights provided by various experts, a lot of preventive measures need to be taken. It is all about having the right ingredients and taking them in the correct proportion. In this very chapter, I am going to share the secrets about the proactive measures that need to be taken to protect yourself and the finest procedure of creating your sanitizer with the ingredients you might already be having at home.

Make Sure You Have the Right Ingredients

The breakneck transmission of COVID-19 has made the people spur to prepare their sanitizer recipes. Although it seems easy, you need to follow the exact procedure, the very right proportions of the ingredients and, most importantly, the truest ingredients to make one. You are wished to have valid information on methods that are being followed to make such products so that you do not harm your skin while making it. As specified by several disease professionals, it is not an atrocious idea to make sanitizers at home only if you can measure the appropriate quantity of isopropyl alcohol.

While it is very important to toss out germs by washing as frequently as it is required to stop the coronavirus from spreading, it is difficult for many of us to be around soap, sink, and water all the time or to just rush to the nearest pharmacy only to find unfilled shelves. What we can do to avoid such circumstances is to prepare DIY sanitizer for ourselves. It may seem harder but not impossible. So, here I am listing down the correct ingredients to start with.

The process is very easy to learn and quite simple because all you require are two ingredients that are crucial for preparing a persuasive product.

- The first ingredient you will require is aloe vera gel. It is an essential plant that is being used by the pharmaceuticals globally. The water-filled tissues in the leaves of the plant are considered as the gelatinous substance, which is known to contain several helpful compounds including vitamins, amino acids, antioxidants, and minerals. It also is known to contain antioxidants belonging to an extensive family known as polyphenols helps to stop the growth of bacteria. Although this gel does not compensate for killing this deadly virus (COVID-19), it does make sure that our hands are moisturized and in good condition while we are using this solution.

- The second ingredient that we will be using is isopropyl alcohol. Isopropyl alcohol is known to contain about ninety-nine percent of alcohol. This is the most important ingredient for making this sanitizer. This is because it is efficient in breaking the protein of this virus by forming new hydrogen bonds instead of the protein flanking chains of the virus and new alcohol molecules.

Ethanol is very much effective in killing viruses. It has been in use since the late 1800s. Most sanitizers, which are alcohol-based, have been made after combining with ethanol. We have already been introduced to the deceasing property of this ingredient from the cases of MERS and SARS. Still, you need to keep this in your mind that simply splashing ethanol on your hand will not kill the virus. You will have to cover your hands with this solution by rubbing throughout, in between the fingers and getting underneath the fingernails to kill any abiding germs.

Your Home Bar Cannot Be Used For Making Sanitizer

The proportion of alcohol you will be using to prepare your hand sanitizer requires to be at 180 proof mark (or 90 % alcohol). Considering a proportion of alcohol lower than this will not do any help as you will be eventually mixing it with aloe vera gel, which will ultimately be decreasing the potency of the alcohol. We all understand the fact that an effective sanitizer is exactly what we should have created to protect ourselves against the coronavirus (COVID-19). You might even think that the distilled spirit that is kept on your liquor chiffonier will be utilized as a substitute for 90% alcohol, which will not work here. Whiskey, rum, or even vodka won't develop a beneficial sanitizer because their alcohol content runs around a proof mark of 80 or 40% and, therefore, they will not be able to kill an enveloped virus-like a corona.

What alcohol does to the bacteria is that they either poison their cells or prevent the bacteria to get the nutrients it needs. It helps to burst the cell membrane of bacteria and viruses by its strength. But, whether you are using vodka or rum or whiskey, it will be just a waste as a sanitizing ingredient. Vodkas have about 40 % of alcohol content, which is just not up to the mark for killing a devastating virus-like a corona. Contrarily, ethanol, which has an alcohol content of about 90 % or a proof mark of 180, is highly efficient in destroying the outer envelope of Coronavirus.

Mix the Ingredients in the Right Proportion

The making of a successful and effective sanitizer comes with the mixing of two ingredients (isopropyl alcohol and gel of aloe vera plant) in the exact proportion as it is required to. A precise measurement of the ingredients is very much essential for the product to become operative. Incorrect analysis of the ingredients being used can do more harm to your body than the good. It can lead to severe irritations and skin problems. Therefore, you should avoid making a solution that is weak to denature the protein coat of the virus and a solution strong for your skin to handle the strength.

The recipe that I am going to write down will be containing an alcohol content of approximately sixty-one percent (which has been proven to be the exact concentration required to transform the virus protein, which is even more fast and effective than alcohol that is 99 percent by volume). However, if you want to create a sanitizer that has got higher alcohol content, you simply need to reduce the quantity of aloe gel in your solution to a quarter cup as it is found to ease down the burning sensation of alcohol.

- The first thing you need to do is measure out a one-third cup of the gel of aloe vera and about a two-third cup of ninety-nine percent of isopropyl alcohol.
- Take a small-sized bowl and add both the substances to it. Mix these two ingredients by whipping and combine until they mix up well.
- You need to add volatile oil to the solution to give a sweet fragrance to it, reducing the strong smell of alcohol. Add about three to five drops of oil to the bowl and mix.
- You can use a clean and empty bottle of hand sanitizer or even a bottle of travel shampoo and discharge the mixture you have just prepared into it.
- After you are completed with pouring the solution into a bottle, allow it to sit for about seventy-two hours. It will help by killing any bacteria that might have been introduced while preparing the solution (as recommended by WHO).

Use the Sanitizer in the Right Manner

It is not just about using a hand sanitizer randomly but the correct manner and the identical time of using it. Hand sanitizers are of course being marketed on a large scale to deal with germs specifically during a tough situation like this when people are on their verge of safeguarding themselves from the coronavirus. But at the same time, it is also important to know when you need to call for the sanitizer. It is as well important to discern when it is crucial to use a precautionary solution and when it is only useful, categorically, when we are dealing with a period of scarcity.

- While the sanitizer we have prepared has an alcohol content that is strong enough to denature the envelope of the virus, it is not that much effective in killing viruses without an envelope or bacterial spores.

- At the same time, hand sanitizers are productive only when they are clean and grease-free. The sanitizers are more likely to work in clinical settings like nursing homes and hospitals where the hands are not heavily spoiled. Some of the researches have proved that the sanitizers may work to some extent on specific germs on slightly greasy hands. But when we are in a community setting, surrounded by many people and doing a lot of activities, such as playing various types of sport, working in the garden, fishing or handling food the hand sanitizer will not show its effect.

- The hand sanitizer must be applied all over the palm in a procedure that has been simplified by the CDC. It instructs you to cover the surface of both hands with the sanitizer you have prepared and keep rubbing until it has dried up on your skin.

- In the end, hand sanitizers are recommended to use when soaps and water are inaccessible. Washing with soap mechanically helps in removing all types of chemicals, dirt, germs, and grease. You should always try to clean both hands with water and soap and store sanitizers for an emergency, whatever may be the situation.

Disinfecting vs. Sanitizing

We often get confused with the two terms – disinfecting and sanitizing. We lean towards using these terms interchangeably. But let me break the ice. There is certainly a legal distinction between the two. For instance, you are cooking and there is food spill all over your kitchen slab and now you are required to decide on the method and product that you use to do away with conceivably hazardous germ and dirt. What will you do? Will you disinfect or sanitize? For that, you are required to know the characteristics of both disinfectants and sanitizers. Here, I will be providing you with the same.

Disinfectant

These are agents that are used to destroy and inactivate microorganisms on the inert surfaces. It is not powerful in killing all kinds of life and it is less compelling than sanitization. It is not effective in killing spores of bacteria that are resistant, which, otherwise, is effectively done by sanitizers. Disinfectants mainly work by damaging the cell membrane of different microbes (though not all) or by interfering with metabolism. But, they work on a wide range of destroying more germs than sanitizers and therefore, they are used time and again in hospitals, bathrooms, kitchens, and during surgeries to decease infectious organisms.

Sanitizer

Sanitizers are liquid or gel-like agents that are believed to destroy about 99.99 percent of bacterial spores within thirty seconds. Sanitizers are the most effective when it comes to killing *norovirus* because of the presence of isopropyl alcohol in it. Rubbing your hands with alcohol-based sanitizers proves to be extremely potent in disrupting the enveloped viruses like coronavirus, flu virus, HIV and common cold virus. It effectively kills all types of life.

Chapter 4: Benefits of Making Your Own Sanitizer

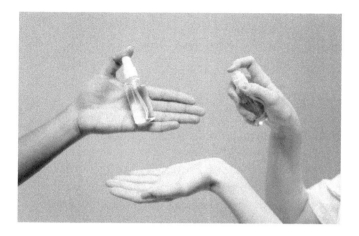

Washing your hands with hand sanitizers are an effective and convenient way of cleaning your hands when soap and water are not available. The most vital ingredient required to make sanitizer is alcohol. Sanitizers containing more than 60 percent of alcohol are most effective in killing bacteria and germs. The accepted versions of alcohol in alcohol-based hand sanitizers are ethanol, isopropyl alcohol, and propanol.

Nowadays, American lives can be pretty much summed up by-products in the supermarket being replaced by mass panic and everyone looking for means to protect themselves. COVID-19 has proved that it's no joke, so it's essential that we put in extra effort to save ourselves and everyone around us. While there's still no vaccine or cure available, studies have proven that the virus can be killed by washing our hands frequently with soap and water or using a hand sanitizer. However, you can hardly find any hand sanitizers in stores. So, why not make your own hand sanitizer at home.

Advantages of Making Sanitizers At Home

Little organizations are also turning their models up and started delivering hand sanitizers. A locally situated organization has its essential office situated inside the proprietor's house. In order to make a business home business, you just have to work from premises similar to the ones you live in rather than purchasing a house. Although we generally expect locally situated entrepreneurs to work from home, it isn't generally the case.

- **Private freedom:** If you are accustomed to wasting hours in the gridlock of rush hours, coming and going to work, beginning a locally situated organization can provide you with two energizing advantages – recovering the lost time and a freshly discovered autonomy. According to the US, a normal American spends about 348 hours driving every year. Starting a locally situated business can provide you with some additional hours to regain control of your own life. Moreover, there are no supervisors, no fixed time of work, no clothing restrictions, and no flexibility agency government issues. The capacity to oversee time, close to home inspiration, and consistency is all you need. You also get to keep the cash that you are earning. It is a golden rule that the harder you work, the more you can earn. You don't have to sit tight, waiting for a promotion or raise. Your outcomes are directly related to your capability of winning. You work more and convey better. You'll also save cash required for gas and nourishment. Arranging lunch from home is more practical and it also lets you take a decent break during the workday.

- **Increase potential:** Beginning your own locally situated business with a large number of organizations and parts means that you can create your own salary delivering openings. Great job opportunities can be rare in specific areas. Limited-time motivators are also decreasing in significant organizations.

- **Less threat:** You need even less money for a new business than an establishment or any unattached business if you run a business from home. Moreover, when your organization is ready to take action, looking over it is less expensive and less difficult than organizing it from a different place.

- **Duty motivators:** When you get your home and your office under one roof, there is a scope of tax cuts. You can also deduct a part of the working and deterioration costs as organization costs. It can be a level of your annual charges, home loan, power, protection, and family upkeep costs.

- **Less fatigue:** When you work from home, you can juggle the weights of work and family more easily as you can set your own timetable.

You may have to perform the role of deals chief, administrator of business development, expert, advertising authority and many more. This involves you with all the aspects of running an organization and thereby makes you attract much more.

- **An inventive springboard:** Starting your office from home can open a door for you to place your interests and inclinations into being, helping you to make money for your imaginative abilities.

- **Developing productivity:** You will get more free time now that you don't need to spend time and energy on driving or trivial gatherings. You can use the time and energy to make the accomplishment of your organization.

Keep Yourself Clean Using Reliable Sources

The pH of any great skin is about 5.5, which is slightly acidic. Most conventional hand sanitizers have a higher pH, about as high as 11. If the pH of the body is very high, the body will retaliate and re-establish its ordinary pH by delivering overabundance sebum. Nonetheless, the dangerous pH is protected by the build-up from sanitizers. The skin may become excessively slick. Moreover, the build-up from the sanitizers emulsifies the lipid framework of the skin. However, if you make your own sanitizer, you can make it according to your own requirements. It will assist you with cleaning your hand and keep you solid as well.

Therefore, the benefits of making your own hand sanitizers can be summed up as:

- You know and can control the ingredients that you want to add to your sanitizer. You don't have to worry about the potentially harmful chemicals that are added to commercially made sanitizers labeled as "fragrance."

- You can choose to add whatever scents that you want. Enjoy a little aromatherapy while warding off germs.

- You can add some aloe vera gel into your hand sanitizer. It acts as a moisturizing agent so your hands won't get dried out when you use the sanitizer. This is a common complaint about commercially made hand sanitizers.

- The ingredients that are left over when you finish making your hand sanitizer can be used in other DIY beauty treatments.

- Making your own hand sanitizer will give you the satisfaction of knowing that you made it by yourself.

- Homemade hand sanitizers might even cost you less than buying them from the store, especially in times like these, when you need to use them frequently.

Chapter 5: DIY Sanitizer Recipes

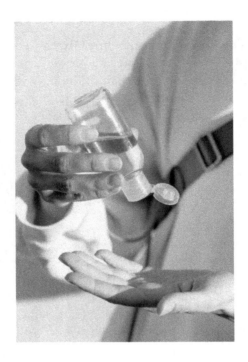

Here is a list of some really easy and super useful sanitizers that you can make at home.

Basic Rubbing Alcohol-Based Sanitizer

Ingredients:

A two-third cup of scouring liquid
A one-third cup of aloe vera gel

Method:

1. Take a glass bowl.
2. Pour the scouring liquid and aloe vera gel into the glass bowl.
3. Blend until both are mixed smoothly.
4. Pour the hand sanitizer through a channel into a small and clean squirt bottle.
5. Store the bottle in a cool place where no direct daylight reaches.
6. Shake the bottle each time smoothly before using the sanitizer.

Hydrogen Peroxide Sanitizer

Ingredients:

One tsp. of glycerin (98%)
One cup of isopropyl alcohol (99%)
One-quarter a cup of sterile water
One tbsp. of hydrogen peroxide (3%)

Method:

1. Take a medium-sized container and use a pouring spout for pouring isopropyl alcohol in the container. Using 99% of alcohol represents almost pure alcohol.
2. Mix hydrogen peroxide in the container with isopropyl alcohol.
3. Then, add glycerin to the mixture and continue stirring with a clean spoon to mix all ingredients in the mixture. It will take more time as the thickness of glycerin is more compared to hydrogen peroxide or isopropyl alcohol. If the container is facilitated with a lid, you can close the lid after adding ingredients. Shake the container to mix them well.
4. Pour the sterile water in the container after measuring it.
5. Sanitize the empty bottles by spraying with the remaining alcohol. Leave the bottles sometimes to evaporate the alcohol. Then, pour the prepared sanitizer in the bottles.
6. Label the bottle to identify as the bottles with sanitizer.

Note: You can use boiled after cooling instead of sterile water.

Aloe Vera Gel Sanitizer

Ingredients:

Half-cup of aloe vera gel (natural)
One cup of isopropyl alcohol (91%)
Fifteen drops of tea tree oil

Method:

1. Use a medium-sized container for taking isopropyl alcohol with the help of a pouring spout.
2. Measure aloe vera gel and combine it in the container with alcohol. The presence of aloe vera will help to maintain the smoothness of your hands, providing protection against the bad effect of alcohol.
3. Mix tea tree oil in the mixture.
4. Make a homogeneous gel by stirring or whisking the mixture.
5. Take the bottles which will be used for keeping prepared hand sanitizer.
   Spray the remaining isopropyl alcohol to sanitize the bottles. Leave them to evaporate the alcohol completely. Then, use the bottles for pouring prepared hand sanitizer.
6. Stick the label to the bottles containing hand sanitizer for identifying them.

Note: You can buy aloe vera from the shop for making hand sanitizer. Then, it will take a little more time to be absorbed within your hands. The reason is that the hand sanitizer made up with natural aloe vera is stickier than the hand sanitizer made up with store-bought aloe vera. Moreover, you can use other essential oils such as lemongrass, lavender, eucalyptus, etc. which act as antibacterial.

Lemon Sanitizer

Ingredients:

One cup of 70% alcohol
Ten drops of tea tree essential oil
Ten drops of lemon essential oil

Method:

1. Use a sterilized glass jar or container.
2. Pour alcohol into the jar.
3. Add ten drops of lemon essential oil into the jar.
4. Stir well with a sterile glass-made stick and mix the solution.
5. Add ten drops of tea tree essential oil into the solution and again stir until the solution gets smooth.
6. Pour the lemon sanitizer into the sterile bottles or dispenser.

Lavender and Tea Tree Oil Sanitizer

Ingredients:

Five drops of tea tree oil
Two cups of water (bubbled and cooled)
Two tbsps. of scouring liquor
Twenty drops of basic lavender oil
Half a tbsp. of aloe vera gel

Method:

1. Take a glass bowl for mixing scouring liquor, basic lavender oil, and tea tree oil. Stir the mixture to combine well.
2. Mix aloe vera gel in the mixture and combine the ingredients completely.
3. Then, add water to the mixture and stir it to make a homogeneous mixture.
4. Pour the prepared hand sanitizer in clean squirt bottles by using the channel.
5. Protect the bottles from direct sunlight and store them in a cool place.
6. It is essential to shake well the bottles before using it.

Orange Sanitizer

Ingredients:

One cup Isopropyl alcohol (99.8%)
A quarter cup of sterile, distilled water
One tbsp. hydrogen peroxide (3%)
Five drops of orange essential oil

Method:

1. Take a sterilized glass container.
2. Pour Isopropyl alcohol into the container.
3. Pour hydrogen peroxide into the jar and mix both with a sterile glass stick.
4. Pour distilled water into the mixture and stir again for mixing uniformly.
5. Add five drops of orange essential oil and continue stirring to prepare a homogenous mixture.
6. Channelize the sanitizer into the sterile bottles or dispensers.
7. Finally, fix the label mentioning the ingredients on the bottles or dispensers.

Eucalyptus Oil Sanitizer

Ingredients:

Ten drops eucalyptus oil (basic)
Two-third a cup of scouring liquor
One-third a cup of aloe vera gel

Method:

1. Use a glass bowl for mixing basic eucalyptus oil and scouring liquor. Stir the mixture to combine them well.
2. Then, mix aloe vera gel in the mixture and stir it to make a homogeneous mixture.
3. Take clean squirt bottles and use the channel for pouring prepared hand sanitizer in these bottles.
4. Store these bottles in a cool place to avoid direct sunlight.
5. It is essential to shake the hand sanitizer properly before using it.

Green Apple Sanitizer

Ingredients:

One cup of 70% alcohol vodka
Ten drops of tea tree oil
Ten drops of green apple essential oil

Method:

1. Use a sterile glass jar.
2. Pour 70% alcohol vodka into the jar.
3. Pour ten drops of tea tree oil into a jar and stir well until both mixes uniformly.
4. Pour ten drops of green apple essential oil and again stir well to form a homogenous mixture.
5. The sanitizer is ready and you have to channelize it into the sterilized bottles or dispensers.
6. In the end, label the bottles or dispensers with the ingredients used to prepare the sanitizer.

Grapefruit Sanitizer

Ingredients:

Half-cup Isopropyl alcohol (99%)
A one-third cup sterile, distilled water
Ten drops of grapefruit essential oil

Method:

1. Sterilize a glass jar to prepare sanitizer.
2. Pour 99% Isopropyl alcohol into the jar.
3. Pour sterile, distilled water into the jar, and stir well so that both mix uniformly.
4. Pour ten drops of grapefruit essential oil and stir again uniformly so that the mixture gets homogenous.
5. Your sanitizer is ready to channelize it into the sterilized bottles or dispensers.
6. Finally, label the bottles or dispensers with the composition of ingredients used to prepare the sanitizer.

Tea Tree and Eucalyptus Oil Sanitizer

Ingredients:

One tbsp. of scouring liquor
Fifteen drops of basic eucalyptus oil
Two cups of water (bubbled and cooled)
Five drops of tea tree oil
Half a tbsp. of aloe vera gel

Method:

1. Use a glass bowl for mixing tea tree oil, basic eucalyptus oil, and scouring liquor. Stir the mixture to combine them well.
2. Combine aloe vera gel in the bowl with mixture and stir it for mixing all the ingredients.
3. Then, stir the mixture after adding bubbled and cooled water in the bowl and make a homogeneous mixture.
4. Pour the prepared hand sanitizer in clean squirt bottles by using the channel.
5. Store the bottles in a cool place with the protection of direct sunlight.
6. It is important to shake the hand sanitizer thoroughly before using it.

Peppermint Oil Sanitizer

Ingredients:

One tbsp. of scouring liquid
Two cups of sterile distilled water
Fifteen drops of basic peppermint oil
Half tbsp. aloe vera gel
Five drops of tea tree oil

Method:

1. Take a sterile glass bowl.
2. Pour scouring liquid, fifteen drops peppermint basic oil, and five drops tea tree oil into the bowl.
3. Stir the components with a sterile glass stick until the components mix well.
4. Add half tbsp. aloe vera gel and stir again until the solution gets smooth.
5. Now pour two cups of sterile water and continue stirring until the mixture gets homogenous.
6. Then, pour the sanitizer into the sterilized squirt bottles through a channel.
7. Store in a cool place where daylight cannot reach.
8. Gently shake the bottle before use.

Orange and Tea Tree Oil Sanitizer

Ingredients:

One tbsp. of scouring liquid
Two cups of bubbled and finally cooled water
Five drops of orange fundamental oil
Half tbsp. aloe vera gel
Five drops of tea tree oil

Method:

1. Pour scouring liquid, orange fundamental oil, and five drops of tea tree oil into a sterilized glass bowl.
2. Stir the components until everything mixes well.
3. Add aloe vera gel and stir further until the solution gets smooth.
4. Now pour sterile water and continue stirring until the mixture becomes homogeneous.
5. Sanitizer is ready and pours it into the sterilized squirt bottles through a pipe.
6. Store in a cool place away from direct daylight.
7. Gently shake the bottle before use.

Lavender Sanitizer

Ingredients:

Eight to ten drops of basic lavender oil
Half a tbsp. of aloe vera gel
Two-third a cup of scouring liquor

Method:

1. Take a glass bowl and mix basic lavender oil with scouring liquor in the bowl. Stir the mixture to combine them well.
2. Then, combine aloe vera gel in the mixture and stir it to mix all the ingredients completely.
3. Use clean squirt bottles for storing prepared hand sanitizer. Also, use the channel for pouring hand sanitizer into squirt bottles.
4. Keep the bottles protected from direct sunlight and store them in a cool place.
5. Don't forget to shake the bottles of hand sanitizer thoroughly before sanitizing your hands.

Orange and Cinnamon Sanitizer

Ingredients:

A three-fourth cup of scouring liquid
Two cups of bubbled and finally cooled water
Ten drops of sweet orange oil
A quarter cup of aloe vera gel
Ten drops of cinnamon fundamental oil
A one-eighth cup of vegetable glycerin

Method:

1. Put scouring liquid, orange oil, and cinnamon fundamental oil into a sterilized glass bowl, and stir well.
2. Add aloe vera gel and vegetable glycerin and stir further until everything consolidates smoothly.
3. Now, add sterile water and continue stirring until the mixture becomes homogeneous.
4. Now fill the sterilized squirt bottles by sanitizer through a pipe.
5. Store in a cool place away from direct daylight.
6. Gently shake the bottle before use.

Lime Oil Sanitizer

Ingredients:

One tbsp. of scouring liquid
Two cups of boiled and cooled water
Five drops of lime basic oil
Half tbsp. of aloe vera gel
Five drops of tea tree oil

Method:

1. Put scouring liquid, lime basic oil, and tea tree oil into a sterilized glass bowl and stir well.
2. Add aloe vera gel and stir further until everything mixes smoothly.
3. Now, add sterile water and continue stirring until the mixture gets uniform.
4. Now fill the sterilized squirt bottles by lime oil sanitizer through a pipe.
5. Store in a cool place away from direct daylight.
6. Gently shake the bottle each time before use.

Vitamin E and Sweet Orange Sanitizer

Ingredients:

Ten drops of sweet orange oil
Two tsps. aloe vera gel
Two tsps. Vitamin E oil
One tbsp. ethyl liquor
One cup of boiled and cooled water

Method:

1. Pour ethyl liquor, Vitamin E oil, and sweet orange oil into a sterile glass bowl and stir well.
2. Add aloe vera gel and stir again until all components mix smoothly.
3. Now, add sterile water and continue stirring until the mixture gets homogeneous.
4. Now fill the sterilized dispensers with sanitizer through a channel.
5. Store dispensers in a place away from direct sunlight.
6. Gently shake the bottle each time before use.

Cinnamon And Lemongrass Oil Sanitizer

Ingredients:

Ten drops of cinnamon fundamental oil
Five drops of lemongrass fundamental oil
Ten drops of tea tree oil
A quarter cup of aloe vera gel
Half tsp. vegetable glycerin
One tbsp. scouring liquor

Method:

1. Pour scouring liquor, cinnamon fundamental oil, lemongrass fundamental oil, and tea tree oil into a sterile glass bowl and stir well.
2. Add aloe vera gel and vegetable glycerin into the bowl and stir again until all components mix smoothly.
3. Now fill the sterilized dispensers with sanitizer through a channel.
4. Store dispensers in a place away from direct sunlight.
5. Gently shake the bottle each time before use.

Cardamom Sanitizer

Ingredients:

Fifteen drops of cardamom basic oil
Five drops of tea tree oil
Half tbsp. of aloe vera gel
One tbsp. scouring liquor
Two cups of sterilized water

Method:

1. Pour scouring liquor, cardamom basic oil, tea tree oil into a sterilized glass bowl and stir well with a sterile glass stick.
2. Add aloe vera gel and blend everything in a way so that all components mix smoothly.
3. Now, pour sterile water and stir again until the solution gets homogeneous.
4. Cardamom sanitizer is ready to pour it in the sterilized dispensers through a pipe.
5. Keep dispensers in a shaded place to avoid direct sunlight.
6. Gently shake the bottle each time before use.

Chamomile Sanitizer

Ingredients:

One tbsp. of scouring liquor
Fifteen drops of basic chamomile oil
Two cups of water (bubbled and cooled)
Five drops of tea tree oil
Half a tbsp. of aloe vera gel

Method:

1. Make a mixture using scouring liquor, basic chamomile oil, and tea tree oil in a glass bowl. Stir the to combine well.
2. Mix aloe vera gel in the glass bowl with the mixture and stir it to combine well.
3. Now, add water and blend with the mixture to make a homogeneous solution.
4. Use a channel to transfer prepared hand sanitizer into clean spray bottles.
5. Place the bottles in a cool place for storing and maintain protection from the sunlight.
6. Don't forget to shake well the bottles before using the hand sanitizer.

Rose Sanitizer

Ingredients:

Ten drops of tea tree oil
One cup of alcohol vodka (70%)
A one-quarter tbsp. of vitamin E oil
Ten drops of rose oil

Method:

1. Sterilize a container and mix alcohol vodka and tea tree oil in the container.
2. Then, combine vitamin E oil and pure rose oil in the container with the mixture. Stir it to combine all the ingredients of the mixture completely.
3. Use a sterile spray bottle or dispenser to store the prepared hand sanitizer.
4. Keep the bottle or dispenser with hand sanitizer in a cool place and also maintain protection from the sunlight to avoid any direct exposure.

Note: Generally, people love the scent of rose. For this reason, rose oil is used as an ingredient for making commercial hand sanitizers.

Jasmine Sanitizer

Ingredients:

Ten drops of essential oil (Jasmine)
A two-third cup of alcohol vodka (70%)
A quarter tbsp. of vitamin E oil
Five tbsps. of witch hazel

Method:

1. Take a sterile container and use it to make a mixture of alcohol vodka, Jasmine essential oil, witch hazel, and vitamin E oil. Stir the mixture to combine well.
2. Sterilize the spray bottle or dispenser and use it for pouring the prepared hand sanitizer.
3. Store the bottle or dispenser with hand sanitizer in a cool place, protecting from the daylight.

Note: Jasmine essential oil is used to prepare hand sanitizer due to its antimicrobial properties. It also helps to keep smooth your hand skin after using hand sanitizer.

Caraway Sanitizer

Ingredients:

One tbsp. of scouring liquid
Two cups of bubbled and cooled water
Five drops of caraway basic oil
Half tbsp. of aloe vera gel
Five drops of tea tree oil

Method:

1. Pour scouring liquid, tea tree oil, and caraway basic oil into a sterilized glass bowl and stir well.
2. Add aloe vera gel and stir further until everything mixes smoothly.
3. Now, add sterile water and continue stirring until the mixture gets uniform.
4. Now fill the sterilized squirt bottles by sanitizer through a pipe.
5. Keep the bottles in a shaded place.
6. Gently shake the bottle before use.

Fennel Sanitizer

Ingredients:

Five drops of fennel basic oil
Five drops of tea tree oil
Half tbsp. of aloe vera gel
One tbsp. of scouring liquor
Two cups of boiled and cooled water

Method:

1. Take a sterile glass bowl.
2. Pour fennel basic oil, tea tree oil, and scouring liquor into the bowl and stir well with a sterile glass stick.
3. Pour aloe vera gel and stir again.
4. Pour sterile water into the mixture and stir again for mixing uniformly.
5. Channelize the sanitizer into the sterile bottles or dispensers.
6. Store bottles in a shaded, cool place.
7. Gently shake the bottle each time before use.

Lychee Sanitizer

Ingredients:

One cup Isopropyl alcohol (99.8%)
One tbsp. hydrogen peroxide (3%)
Quarter cup sterilized, distilled water
Five drops of lychee essential oil

Method:

1. You need to collect a glass jar, a glass-made stirring stick, and bottles to fill sanitizer. All of these must be sterilized before use.
2. Pour the Isopropyl alcohol into a glass jar and add hydrogen peroxide into it.
3. Stir well with stirring stick until both mixed smoothly.
4. Pour sterile water in the mixture and stir again.
5. Add lychee essential oil and stir the mixture until it gets smooth.
6. Fill the sterilized bottles with the sanitizer through a channel.
7. Mark the bottles of sanitizer, if possible, with a label stating the ingredients used.

Anise Oil Sanitizer

Ingredients:

Five drops of anise basic oil
Five drops of tea tree oil
Half tbsp. of aloe vera gel
One tbsp. of scouring liquor
Two cups of boiled and cooled water

Method:

1. Pour anise basic oil, tea tree oil, and scouring liquor into a sterilized bowl and stir well with a sterile glass stick.
2. Pour aloe vera gel and stir again to mix properly.
3. Add sterile water into the mixture and stir again for mixing the solution uniformly.
4. Channelize the sanitizer into the sterile bottles or dispensers.
5. Store the bottles in a shaded, cool place.
6. Shake the bottle gently each time before use.

Balsam Fir Oil Sanitizer

Ingredients:

Fifteen drops of resin fir fundamental oil
Five drops of tea tree oil
Half tbsp. of aloe vera gel
One tbsp. of scouring liquor
Two cups of bubbled and cooled water

Method:

1. You need to collect a glass bowl, a glass-made stirring stick, and bottles to fill sanitizer. All these must be sterilized before use.
2. Pour the resin fir fundamental oil, tea tree oil, and scouring liquor into the glass bowl.
3. Stir well until all three mix smoothly.
4. Add aloe vera gel and stir again to get a well-consolidated mixture.
5. Pour sterile water in the mixture and stir again until the solution gets homogenous.
6. Fill the sterilized bottles with the sanitizer through a channel.
7. Store the bottles in a shaded, cool place.
8. Shake the bottle gently every time before using the sanitizer.

Ylang Ylang Sanitizer

Ingredients:

One tbsp. of hydrogen peroxide (3%)
A one-quarter cup of water (sterile and distilled)
Ten drops of essential oil (Ylang Ylang)
One cups of isopropyl alcohol (99.8%)

Method:

1. Use a clean container to make a mixture of isopropyl alcohol and hydrogen peroxide. Stir the mixture to mix well.
2. Combine sterile and distilled water and Ylang Ylang essential oil to the mixture. Mix all the ingredients thoroughly.
3. Transfer the prepared hand sanitizer to a sterile spray bottle.
4. Store the bottle with sanitizer in a cool atmosphere avoiding the sunlight.

Note: Ylang Ylang has a component named linalool, which acts as an antifungal and antibacterial agent.

Lemongrass Sanitizer

Ingredients:

Five tbsp. of witch hazel
A one-quarter tbsp. of vitamin E oil
A two-third cup of alcohol vodka (70%)
Ten drops of essential oil (lemongrass)

Method:

1. Use a clean glass bowl to mix alcohol vodka with witch hazel.
2. Then, combine vitamin E oil and lemongrass essential oil in the glass bowl with the mixture. Stir the mixture for thoroughly mixing all the ingredients in it.
3. Use sterile dispenser for transferring the prepared hand sanitizer.
4. Place the dispenser with hand sanitizer in a cool area for avoiding the direct sunlight.

Note: Use of lemongrass essential oil in hand sanitizer includes minty scent within it. Lemongrass acts as an antimicrobial agent according to its property.

Frankincense Sanitizer

Ingredients:

Five drops of frankincense fundamental oil
Five drops of tea tree oil
Half tbsp. of aloe vera gel
One tbsp. of scouring liquor
Two cups of bubbled and cooled water

Method:

1. Arrange a glass bowl, a glass-made stirring stick, and bottles to fill sanitizer. Get all these sterilized before use.
2. Pour the frankincense fundamental oil, tea tree oil, and scouring liquor into the glass bowl and stir well to mix all components smoothly.
3. Add aloe vera gel and stir again to get a well-consolidated mixture.
4. Pour sterile water in the mixture and stir again until the solution gets homogenous.
5. Fill the sterilized bottles with the sanitizer through a channel.
6. Store the bottles in a shaded, cool place.
7. Shake the bottle gently every time before using the sanitizer.

Vanilla Sanitizer

Ingredients:

Fifteen drops of vanilla fundamental oil
Five drops of tea tree oil
Half tbsp. of aloe vera gel
One tbsp. of scouring liquor
Two cups of bubbled and cooled water

Method:

1. Arrange sterilized glass bowl, glass-made stirring stick, and bottles to fill sanitizer.
2. Pour the vanilla fundamental oil, tea tree oil, and scouring liquor into the glass bowl and stir well to mix all ingredients properly.
3. Add aloe vera gel and stir again to get a well-mixed solution.
4. Pour water in the mixture and stir again until the solution gets homogenous.
5. Fill the sterilized bottles with the sanitizer through a channel.
6. Store the bottles in a shaded, cool place.
7. Shake the bottle gently every time before using the sanitizer.

Calamus Oil Sanitizer

Ingredients:

One tbsp. of scouring liquid
Two cups of boiled and cooled water
Five drops of calamus fundamental oil
Half tbsp. of aloe vera gel
Five drops of tea tree oil

Method:

1. Pour scouring liquid, calamus fundamental oil, and tea tree oil into a sterilized glass bowl and stir well.
2. Add aloe vera gel and stir further until everything mixes smoothly.
3. Now, add sterile water and continue stirring until the mixture gets uniform.
4. Now fill the sterilized squirt bottles by calamus oil sanitizer through a pipe.
5. Store in a cool place away from direct daylight.
6. Gently shake the bottle each time before use.

Calamondin Oil Sanitizer

Ingredients:

Five drops of calamondin fundamental oil
Five drops of tea tree oil
Half tbsp. of aloe vera gel
One tbsp. of scouring liquid
Two cups of boiled and cooled water

Method:

1. Pour tea tree oil, calamus fundamental oil, and scouring liquid into a sterile glass bowl and stir well.
2. Add aloe vera gel and stir further until everything gets smooth.
3. Now, add sterile water and continue stirring until the mixture gets uniform.
4. Now fill the sterilized squirt bottles by calamondin oil sanitizer through a pipe.
5. Store in a cool place away from direct daylight.
6. Gently shake the bottle each time before use.

Davana Oil Sanitizer

Ingredients:

One tbsp. of scouring liquid
Five drops of davana basic oil
Half tbsp. of aloe vera gel
Five drops of tea tree oil
Two cups of boiled and cooled water

Method:

1. Pour davana basic oil, scouring liquid, and tea tree oil into a sterilized glass bowl and stir well.
2. Add aloe vera gel and stir again until all ingredients mix smoothly.
3. Now, add sterile water and continue stirring until the mixture gets homogeneous.
4. Now fill the sterilized squirt bottles with davana oil sanitizer through a pipe.
5. Store in a cool place away from direct daylight.
6. Gently shake the bottle each time before use.

Patchouli Sanitizer

Ingredients:

Twenty drops of patchouli essential oil
A half-cup of aloe vera gel
One cup of isopropyl alcohol (70-99.8%)
Quarter tbsp. Vitamin E oil

Method:

1. Arrange for sterile dispensers, a glass-made stirring stick, a glass bowl for preparing the sanitizer.
2. Pour patchouli essential oil and Vitamin E oil into the glass bowl and stir well to mix the ingredients uniformly.
3. Add aloe vera gel and isopropyl alcohol into the bowl.
4. Stir again to get a homogeneous mixture.
5. Sanitizer is ready and you can fill the dispensers with the sanitizer through a channel.
6. Fix a label on the dispensers stating the ingredients.
7. Store the dispensers in a shaded place to avoid direct daylight.
8. Gently shake the dispenser each time before use.

Galbanum Oil Sanitizer

Ingredients:

Two cups of boiled and cooled water
One tbsp. of scouring liquid
Five drops of tea tree oil
Five drops of galbanum basic oil
Half tbsp. of aloe vera gel

Method:

1. Pour galbanum basic oil, scouring liquid, and tea tree oil into a sterilized glass bowl and stir well.
2. Add aloe vera gel and stir again until all ingredients mix smoothly.
3. Now, add sterile water and keep on stirring until the mixture gets homogeneous.
4. Now fill the sterilized squirt bottles by galbanum oil sanitizer through a channel.
5. Store in a shaded place to maintain room temperature.
6. Gently shake the bottle each time before use.

May Chang Oil Sanitizer

Ingredients:

Five drops of tea tree oil
Five drops of litsea cubeba (scientific name May Chang) basic oil
Two cups of boiled and cooled water
One tbsp. of scouring liquid
Half tbsp. of aloe vera gel

Method:

1. Pour scouring liquid, litsea cubeba fundamental oil, and tea tree oil into a sterilized glass bowl and stir well.
2. Add aloe vera gel and stir further until everything mixes smoothly.
3. Now, add sterile water and further keep on stirring until the mixture gets uniform.
4. Now fill the sterilized squirt bottles by May Chang oil sanitizer through a pipe.
5. Store in a cool place away from direct daylight.
6. Gently shake the bottle each time before use.

Cedarwood Sanitizer

Ingredients:

Twenty drops of cedarwood oil
Half cup aloe vera gel
One cup of isopropyl alcohol (70-99.8%)
Quarter tbsp. of Vitamin E oil

Method:

1. Arrange for a sterilized glass bowl, glass-made stirring stick, and dispensers to fill sanitizer.
2. Add cedarwood oil, isopropyl alcohol into the glass bowl and stir well and observe that both the ingredients mix uniformly.
3. Add aloe vera gel and Vitamin E oil.
4. Stir again and check everything mixes properly.
5. Fill the dispensers with the sanitizer by a pipe.
6. Store the dispensers in a shaded, cool place.
7. Shake the dispenser gently each time before use.

Cypress Sanitizer

Ingredients:

Twenty drops of cypress essential oil
A one-third cup aloe vera gel
A two-third cup of isopropyl alcohol (99.8%)
Quarter tbsp. Vitamin E oil

Method:

1. Arrange for a glass-made stirring stick, sterilized glass bowl, and dispensers to fill sanitizer.
2. Pour cypress essential oil and isopropyl alcohol into the glass bowl and stir well to mix the ingredients smoothly.
3. Add aloe vera gel and Vitamin E oil into the bowl.
4. Stir again to get a homogeneous mixture.
5. Sanitizer is ready and you can fill the dispensers with the sanitizer through a channel.
6. Store the dispensers in a shaded, cool place.
7. Gently shake the dispenser each time before use.

Palmarosa Oil Sanitizer

Ingredients:

Five drops of tea tree oil
Five drops of palmarosa fundamental oil
Two cups of boiled and cooled water
One tbsp. of scouring liquid
Half tbsp. of aloe vera gel

Method:

1. Pour scouring liquid, palmarosa fundamental oil, and tea tree oil into a sterilized glass bowl and stir well.
2. Add aloe vera gel and blend everything to get a smooth mixture.
3. Now, add sterile water and keep on stirring until the mixture gets uniform.
4. Now fill the sterilized squirt bottles by palmarosa oil sanitizer through a pipe.
5. Store in a cool place away from direct daylight.
6. Gently shake the bottle each time before use.

Three-Oils Sanitizer

Ingredients:

Ten drops of lavender basic oil
Twenty drops of tea tree oil
A half tsp. Vitamin E oil
Three tbsps. aloe vera gel
One tbsp. of scouring liquor

Method:

1. Pour scouring liquor, lavender basic oil, and tea tree oil into a sterilized glass bowl and stir well to get a homogenous mixture.
2. Add aloe vera gel and blend to get a smooth mixture.
3. Now, add sterile water and keep on stirring until the mixture gets uniform.
4. Now fill the sterilized squirt bottles by three-oil sanitizer through a pipe.
5. Store in a cool place away from direct daylight.
6. Gently shake the bottle each time before use.

Hyssop Sanitizer

Ingredients:

A half-cup of aloe vera gel
A quarter cup of 70% alcohol vodka
Twenty drops of hyssop essential oil
Quarter tbsp. Vitamin E oil

Method:

1. Arrange for a glass bowl, bottles for filling the sanitizer, and a glass-made stirring stick. Sterilize everything before use.
2. Pour alcohol vodka and aloe vera gel into the glass bowl and stir well to mix the ingredients smoothly.
3. Add hyssop essential oil and Vitamin E oil into the bowl.
4. Stir the solution again to get a homogeneous mixture.
5. Now you can pour the sanitizer into the bottles through a channel.
6. Fix a label on the bottles stating the ingredients.
7. Store the bottles in a shaded place to avoid direct daylight.
8. Gently shake the bottle each time before use.

Vetiver Oil Sanitizer

Ingredients:

Fifteen drops of vetiver basic oil
Five drops of tea tree oil
Half tbsp. of aloe vera gel
One tbsp. of scouring liquor
Two cups of bubbled and cooled water

Method:

1. Take a sterilized glass bowl, glass-made stirring stick, and bottles to fill sanitizer.
2. Pour the vetiver basic oil, tea tree oil, and scouring liquor into the glass bowl and stir everything to mix the ingredients smoothly.
3. Add aloe vera gel and stir again to get a well-mixed solution.
4. Pour water in the mixture and stir again until the solution gets homogenous.
5. Fill the sterilized bottles with the sanitizer through a channel.
6. Store the bottles in a shaded, cool place.
7. Shake the bottle gently every time before using the sanitizer.

Strawberry Sanitizer

Ingredients:

Ten drops of strawberry essential oil
Ten drops of tea tree oil
Half cup aloe vera gel
One cup of 70% alcohol vodka
Quarter tbsp. Vitamin E oil

Method:

1. Take a sterilized glass bowl, glass-made stirring stick, and bottles to fill sanitizer.
2. Put strawberry essential oil, tea tree oil, and Vitamin E oil into the glass bowl and stir everything until the ingredients smoothly.
3. Add aloe vera gel and alcohol vodka.
4. Stir again to get a homogeneous solution.
5. Fill the bottles with the sanitizer through a channel.
6. Store the bottles in a shaded, cool place.

Lavender and Vitamin E Sanitizer

Ingredients:

Five-Ten drops of lavender fundamental oil
Thirty drops of tea tree fundamental oil
Quarter tsp. Vitamin E oil
One oz. of unadulterated aloe vera gel
Three oz. of high-proof vodka

Method:

1. Pour high-proof vodka, lavender fundamental oil, tea tree fundamental oil, and Vitamin E oil into a sterilized glass bowl and stir well until the mixture gets homogenous.
2. Add aloe vera gel and blend well until the mixtures become smooth.
3. Now, through a channel, fill the sterilized squirt bottles by lavender and Vitamin E sanitizer.
4. Store in a cool place away from direct daylight.
5. Gently shake the bottle each time before use.

Four-Oils Sanitizer

Ingredients:

Ten drops of lavender fundamental oil
Twenty drops of tea tree oil
Five drops of lemongrass fundamental oil
One tsp. Vitamin E oil
Two tbsps. aloe vera gel
Four tbsps. of vodka

Method:

1. Take a sterile glass bowl and a glass stir. Pour lavender fundamental oil, lemongrass fundamental oil, and tea tree oil, Vitamin E oil, and vodka into the sterilized glass bowl and stir well until the mixture gets homogenous.
2. Now, add aloe vera gel and blend well all around until the mixture becomes smooth.
3. Your four-oils sanitizer is ready. Now through a channel, fill the sterilized squirt bottles by sanitizer.
4. Store the bottles in a cool place away from direct daylight.
5. Gently shake the bottle each time before use.

Oregano Sanitizer

Ingredients:

Twenty drops of oregano essential oil
A half-cup of aloe vera gel
A quarter cup of 70% alcohol vodka
Quarter tbsp. Vitamin E oil

Method:

1. Arrange for a sterile glass bowl for preparing the sanitizer, dispensers for filling the sanitizer, and a glass-made stirring stick.
2. Pour alcohol vodka and aloe vera gel into the glass bowl and stir well to mix the ingredients uniformly.
3. Add oregano essential oil and Vitamin E oil into the bowl.
4. Stir again to get a homogeneous mixture.
5. Sanitizer is ready and you can fill the dispensers with the sanitizer through a pipe.
6. Fix a label on the dispensers stating the ingredients.
7. Store the dispensers in a shaded place to avoid direct daylight.
8. Gently shake the dispenser each time before use.

Four-Oils and Glycerin Sanitizer

Ingredients:

Two drops of clove bud fundamental oil
Two drops of rosemary fundamental oil
Two drops of eucalyptus fundamental oil
Two drops of cinnamon leaf fundamental oil
A half tsp. vegetable glycerin
One tsp. aloe vera juice
Two tbsps. vodka
Two tbsps. of sterile water

Method:

1. Take a sterile glass bowl and a glass stir. Pour all oils, aloe vera juice, and vodka into the bowl and stir well until the mixture gets homogenous.
2. Now, add vegetable glycerin and blend well until the mixture becomes smooth.
3. Now, pour water and blend further.
4. Your four-oils and glycerin sanitizer is ready. Now, through a channel, fill the sterilized squirt bottles by sanitizer.
5. Store the bottles in a cool place away from direct daylight.
6. Gently shake the bottle each time before use.

Juniper Sanitizer

Ingredients:

Twenty drops of juniper essential oil
A half-cup of aloe vera gel
A cup of isopropyl alcohol (70-99.8%)
Quarter tbsp. Vitamin E oil

Method:

1. Arrange for a glass bowl for preparing the sanitizer, dispensers for filling the sanitizer, and a glass-made stirring stick. Sterilize everything before use.
2. Pour juniper essential oil and Vitamin E oil into the glass bowl and stir well to mix the ingredients smoothly.
3. Add isopropyl alcohol and aloe vera gel into the bowl.
4. Stir the solution again to get a homogeneous mixture.
5. Sanitizer is ready and you can pour it in the dispensers through a pipe.
6. Fix a label on the dispensers stating the ingredients.
7. Store the dispensers in a shaded place to avoid direct daylight.
8. Gently shake the dispenser each time before use.

Turmeric Sanitizer

Ingredients:

One tbsp. of hydrogen peroxide (3%)
A one-quarter cup of water (sterile and distilled)
Ten drops of essential oil (turmeric)
One cup of isopropyl alcohol (99.8%)

Method:

1. Take a sterile glass bowl and combine isopropyl alcohol and hydrogen peroxide in it to make a mixture by stirring them.
2. Also, stir the mixture after mixing turmeric essential oil and sterile and distilled water in the mixture of the glass bowl.
3. Use a channel to pour the prepared hand sanitizer into a sterile spray bottle.
4. Place the hand sanitizer bottle in a cool place and also maintain protection from the heat of the direct sunlight.

Note: Turmeric acts as antibacterial as well as antiviral agent according to its properties. It also helps in healing cuts and injuries.

Cinnamon Sanitizer

Ingredients:

One cup of isopropyl alcohol (99.8%)
Ten drops of essential oil (cinnamon)
One cup of water (sterile and distilled)
One tbsp. of hydrogen peroxide (3%)

Method:

1. Use a clean glass bowl to combine isopropyl alcohol and cinnamon essential oil and stir the mixture for mixing well.
2. Now, mix sterile and distilled water and hydrogen peroxide in the mixture. Stir the mixture until all the ingredients of it mix completely.
3. Then, sterilize a dispenser to pour the prepared cinnamon hand sanitizer. Use a channel to pour the sanitizer into the sterile dispenser.
4. Store the hand sanitizer dispenser in a cool atmosphere to keep away from the sunlight directly.

Note: Cinnamon is used for preparing hand sanitizer due to its antimicrobial property and aromatic scent.

Lemon Balm Sanitizer

Ingredients:

Five tbsp. of witch hazel
Ten drops of essential oil (lemon balm)
A one-quarter tbsp. of vitamin E oil
A two-third cup of alcohol vodka (70%)

Method:

1. Use a clean container for mixing vitamin E oil and alcohol vodka and stir them to combine well.
2. Then, add witch hazel and lemon balm essential oil to the container with the mixture. Mix all the ingredients thoroughly by stirring them.
3. Use a clean spray bottle or dispenser to transfer the prepared lemon balm hand sanitizer.
4. Store the hand sanitizer bottle in a safe and cool place to keep away from the daylight.

Note: Lemon Balm is very effective to fight against viral diseases such as bird flu and influenza due to its antiviral property.

Myrrha Sanitizer

Ingredients:

One cup of isopropyl alcohol (99.8%)
Ten drops of essential oil (Myrrha)
A one-quarter cup of water (sterile and distilled)
One tbsp. of hydrogen peroxide (3%)

Method:

1. Take a clean container and make a mixture with isopropyl alcohol and hydrogen peroxide.
2. Then, combine Myrrha essential oil and sterile and distilled water in the mixture. Stir well to mix all the ingredients completely within the mixture.
3. Use the channel to pour the hand sanitizer from the container into a clean dispenser,
4. Place the hand sanitizer dispenser in a cool place to protect from the sunlight directly.

Note: Myrrha essential oil is used for preparing hand sanitizer as it involves a unique scent within the hand sanitizer. It also acts as an antiviral agent according to its properties.

Clove Sanitizer

Ingredients:

One cup of isopropyl alcohol
Ten drops of essential oil clove)
A one-quarter cup of water (sterile and distilled)
One tbsp. of hydrogen peroxide

Method:

1. Make a mixture of clove essential oil and hydrogen peroxide in a clean glass bowl.
2. Now, mix isopropyl alcohol and sterile and distilled water in the glass bowl. Stir well to combine all the ingredients of the mixture completely.
3. Sterilize squirt bottle to store prepared hand sanitizer. Pour hand sanitizer into the sterile squirt bottle by using a channel.
4. Protect the squirt bottle with hand sanitizer from the heat of the daylight by storing it in a cool atmosphere.

Note: Clove is included within the ingredients of hand sanitizer as it has antiviral properties.

Rosemary Sanitizer

Ingredients:

Ten drops of essential oil (rosemary)
A two-third cup of alcohol vodka (70%)
A one-quarter tbsp. of vitamin E oil
Five tbsps. of witch hazel

Method:

1. Mix alcohol vodka with vitamin E oil in a clean container and Stir the mixture.
2. Then, combine witch hazel and rosemary essential oil in the mixture. Stir the mixture to make a homogeneous mixture of the ingredients.
3. Use a clean squirt bottle to store the hand sanitizer. Also, use a channel for transferring hand sanitizer from the container to the squirt bottle.
4. Place the squirt bottle of hand sanitizer in a cool place to keep away from the sunlight directly.

Note: Rosemary works as an antioxidant and antiviral agent as per its properties. It is used for the treatment of insomnia.

Citronella Sanitizer

Ingredients:

Ten drops of essential oil (citronella)
One cup of isopropyl alcohol (99.8%)
One tbsp. of hydrogen peroxide (3%)
A one-quarter cup of water (sterile and distilled)

Method:

1. Make a mixture by adding isopropyl alcohol and sterile and distilled water in a clean glass bowl.
2. Now, mix citronella essential oil and hydrogen peroxide in the mixture. Stir well for mixing all the ingredients to make a homogeneous solution.
3. Pour the prepared hand sanitizer into a sterile squirt bottle by using a channel.
4. Store the squirt bottle of hand sanitizer in a cool place and keep away from direct sunlight.

Note: Citronella protects to stay safe from the insect. It also works as an antimicrobial agent.

Sage Sanitizer

Ingredients:

A two-third cup of alcohol vodka (70%)
Ten drops of essential oil (sage)
A one-quarter cup of vitamin E oil
Five tbsps. of witch hazel

Method:

1. Use a sterile container to mix witch hazel and sage essential oil. Stir to combine well.
2. Then, add vitamin E oil and alcohol vodka to the container with the mixture. Stir to mix all the ingredients completely.
3. Take the help of a channel to transfer the prepared hand sanitizer into a sterile dispenser from the container.
4. Store the dispenser of hand sanitizer in a cool atmosphere to keep away from the direct sunlight.

Note: Sage essential oil is an agent for healing and soothing as per its properties. It also acts as a natural antimicrobial agent.

Tea Tree Sanitizer

Ingredients:

One cup of isopropyl alcohol (70 to 99.8%)
Twenty drops of tea tree essential oil
Half-cup of aloe vera gel

Method:

1. Sterilize a container and use it for making a mixture of isopropyl alcohol and aloe vera gel. Stir the mixture to combine well.
2. Then, mix tea tree oil in the container. Stir the mixture to combine all the ingredients completely.
3. Transfer the prepared hand sanitizer to a sterile dispenser from the container by using a channel.
4. Store the hand sanitizer dispenser in a cool atmosphere to avoid direct sunlight.
5. Shake well the hand sanitizer dispenser before using it.

Note: Tea tree oil helps to maintain clear skin. It also acts as an antimicrobial agent as per its properties.

Sandalwood Sanitizer

Ingredients:

One tbsp. of scouring liquor
Five drops of sandalwood oil (basic)
Two cups of water (bubbled and cooled)
Five drops of tea tree oil
Half-tbsp. of aloe vera gel

Method:

1. Take a clean glass bowl and make a mixture of scouring liquor, basic sandalwood oil, and tea tree oil in it.
2. Blend the mixture completely after adding aloe vera gel in the mixture.
3. Then, combine bubbled and cooled water in the bowl with the mixture. Stir the mixture to mix all the ingredients thoroughly.
4. Transfer the sandalwood hand sanitizer in a sterile squirt bottle using a channel.
5. Keep the hand sanitizer bottle in a cool place to maintain protection from the sunlight directly.
6. Don't forget to shake well the hand sanitizer bottle before using it.

Note: The basic sandalwood oil involves sandalwood scent and it also has the property to fight against bacteria.

Ginger Oil Sanitizer

Ingredients:

One tbsp. of scouring liquor
Five drops of ginger oil (basic)
Two cups of water (bubbled and cooled)
Five drops of tea tree oil
Half-tbsp. of aloe vera gel

Method:

1. Sterilize a glass bowl and use it for making a mixture of scouring liquor, tea tree oil, and basic ginger oil.
2. Blend well the mixture after adding aloe vera gel in the glass bowl.
3. Add bubbled and cooled water to the mixture and again blend it to combine all the ingredients completely.
4. Sterilize a spray bottle and pour ginger oil sanitizer in it using a channel.
5. Store the spray bottle with sanitizer in a cool place and protect it from direct sunlight.
6. It is important to shake the bottle with sanitizer every time you decide you want to use it.

Note: Ginger acts as an antioxidant and anti-inflammatory agent according to its properties.

Tarragon Oil Sanitizer

Ingredients:

One tbsp. of scouring liquor
Five drops of basic tarragon oil
Two cups of water (bubbled and cooled)
Five drops of tea tree oil
Half-tbsp. of aloe vera gel

Method:

1. Use a clean glass bowl to combine scouring liquor, basic tarragon oil, and tea tree oil and make a mixture.
2. Then, mix aloe vera gel in the glass bowl and combine well in the mixture.
3. Blend the mixture thoroughly after adding bubbled and cooled water to the bowl.
4. Pour the prepared tarragon oil sanitizer in a sterile spray bottle from the glass bowl with the help of a channel.
5. Protect the spray bottle with sanitizer from direct sunlight and place it in a cool place.
6. Shake the sanitizer bottle every time before using it.

Note: Tarragon oil acts as an antibacterial agent according to its properties.

Thyme Oil Sanitizer

Ingredients:

Half-cup of aloe vera gel
A one-quarter cup of scouring liquor
One tbsp. of glycerin (vegetable)
Fifteen to twenty drops of thyme oil (fundamental)

Method:

1. Take a clean glass bowl and use it for making a mixture of fundamental thyme oil and scouring liquor.
2. Blend well the mixture after mixing vegetable glycerin and aloe vera gel in the glass bowl. Make a homogeneous mixture.
3. Use a pipe to transfer the prepared thyme oil sanitizer to a sterile squirt bottle from the glass bowl.
4. Protect the squirt bottle of sanitizer from direct daylight and store it in a cool place.
5. Don't forget to shake the sanitizer bottle thoroughly for each time you decide to use it.

Note: Thyme oil is an active antibacterial and anti-inflammatory agent as per its property.

Pine Oil Sanitizer

Ingredients:

One tbsp. of scouring liquor
Five drops of pine oil (basic)
Two cups of water (bubbled and cooled)
Five drops of tea tree oil
Half-tbsp. of aloe vera gel

Method:

1. Sterilize a glass bowl and use it for mixing scouring liquor, basic pine oil, and tea tree oil.
2. Then, blend the mixture thoroughly after adding aloe vera to the glass bowl.
3. Mix bubbled and cooled water in the mixture and again blend it thoroughly to combine all the ingredients.
4. Now, us a pipe for transferring the prepared pine oil sanitizer to a sterile spray bottle from the glass bowl.
5. Store the spray bottle with sanitizer in a cool place and maintain protection from the direct sunlight.
6. It is essential to shake the sanitizer bottle before the utilization of it.

Note: The basic pine oil is used for the preparation of sanitizer as an active antimicrobial and anti-inflammatory agent as per its properties.

Tsuga Oil Sanitizer

Ingredients:

Half-tbsp. of aloe vera gel
Five drops of tea tree oil
Two cups of water (bubbled and cooled)
Five drops of Tsuga oil (basic)
One tbsp. of scouring liquor

Method:

1. Use a clean glass bowl to prepare a mixture of tea tree oil, basic Tsuga oil, and scouring liquor. Stir the mixture to combine well.
2. Then, combine aloe vera gel in the bowl and stir the mixture again to blend the mixture.
3. Mix bubbled and cooled water in the bowl. Stir the mixture until it becomes a homogeneous mixture.
4. Pour the prepared Tsuga oil sanitizer in a sterile squirt bottle from the bowl through a channel.
5. Store the sanitizer bottle in a cool place and keep away from the direct sunlight.
6. Shake the sanitizer bottle delicately when you decide to use it.

Note: Tsuga oil helps to keep the skin hydrated and supple.

Star Anise Sanitizer

Ingredients:

Half-tbsp. of aloe vera gel
Five drops of tea tree oil
Two cups of water (bubbled and cooled)
Five drops of star anise oil (basic)
One tbsp. of scouring liquor

Method:

1. Make a mixture of tea tree oil, basic star anise oil, and scouring liquor in a clean glass bowl.
2. Combine aloe vera gel in the glass bowl and stir the mixture to blend it within the mixture.
3. Stir well the mixture after adding the water in the bowl and make a homogeneous mixture.
4. Sterilize a dispenser and pour the prepared star anise sanitizer in the sterile dispenser through a channel.
5. Store the dispenser with sanitizer in a cool place and protect it from the sunlight directly.
6. Don't forget to shake delicately the sanitizer bottle before using it.

Note: Star anise oil acts as an antiviral, antibacterial, and antifungal agent according to its properties.

Rosewood Sanitizer

Ingredients:

Half-tbsp. of aloe vera gel
Five drops of tea tree oil
Two cups of water (bubbled and cooled)
Five drops of rosewood oil (fundamental)
One tbsp. of scouring liquor

Method:

1. Sterilize a glass bowl and use it for mixing tea tree oil, scouring liquor, and fundamental rosewood oil.
2. Mix aloe vera gel in the glass bowl and stir the mixture to combine well.
3. Stir the mixture again and make a homogeneous mixture after adding bubbled and cooled water in the bowl.
4. Transfer the prepared rosewood sanitizer to a sterile dispenser through a pipe.
5. Keep away the sanitizer dispenser from the direct sunlight by storing it in a cool place.
6. Shake the sanitizer dispenser delicately when you decide to use it.

Note: Rosewood fundamental oil has a scent to refresh your mind as per its property.

Emil Oil Sanitizer

Ingredients:

Half-tbsp. of aloe vera gel
Five drops of tea tree oil
Two cups of water (bubbled and cooled)
Five drops of Emil oil (fundamental)
One tbsp. of scouring liquor

Method:

1. Use a clean glass bowl for mixing tea tree oil, scouring liquor, and fundamental Emil oil. Stir the mixture to mix them thoroughly.
2. Combine well the mixture after adding aloe vera gel to the glass bowl.
3. Then, mix bubbled and cooled water in the mixture. Stir it to mix all the ingredients completely.
4. Use a channel to pour the prepared Emil oil sanitizer into a clean dispenser from the glass bowl.
5. Protect the sanitizer dispenser from the direct daylight by storing them in a cool place.
6. Shake the sanitizer dispenser thoroughly before using it.

Note: Emil oil is used in sanitizer as it is advantageous for enhancing skin absorption and moisture according to its properties.

Agar Oil Sanitizer

Ingredients:

One tbsp. of scouring liquor
Five drops of agar oil (basic)
Half-tbsp. of aloe vera gel
Five drops of tea tree oil
Two cups of water (bubbled and cooled)

Method:

1. Take a clean glass bowl and make a mixture of tea tree oil, scouring liquor, and basic agar oil. Stir the mixture to mix well.
2. Then, mix aloe vera gel in the glass bowl and stir the mixture again to blend the mixture completely.
3. Add bubbled and cooled water to the glass bowl and blend well the mixture to make a homogeneous solution.
4. Sterilize a spray bottle and transfer the prepared agar oil sanitizer to it from the glass bowl through a channel.
5. Store the spray bottle in a cool place and protect it from direct sunlight.
6. It is essential to shake the spray bottle with sanitizer delicately when you decide to use it.

Note: Agar oil helps to moisturize the skin. It also acts as an antibacterial and antioxidant agent according to its properties.

Fenugreek Sanitizer

Ingredients:

Five drops of tea tree oil
Half-tbsp. of aloe vera gel
Five drops of fenugreek oil (fundamental)
Two cups of water (bubbled and cooled)
One tbsp. of scouring liquor

Method:

1. Use a clean glass bowl to make a mixture of scouring liquor, tea tree oil, and fundamental fenugreek oil. Stir well to mix them thoroughly.
2. Blend the mixture well after adding aloe vera gel in the glass bowl.
3. Combine water in the mixture and blend it completely to make a homogeneous mixture.
4. Use a channel to pour the prepared fenugreek sanitizer in a sterile dispenser from the glass bowl.
5. Place the dispenser with sanitizer in a cool place and keep away from the direct sunlight.
6. Shake the sanitizer dispenser delicately when you use it.

Note: Fenugreek oil acts as an antibacterial, antifungal, and antiviral agent according to its properties.

Balsam of Peru Sanitizer

Ingredients:

Five drops of tea tree oil
Half-tbsp. of aloe vera gel
Five drops of balsam of Perú oil (basic)
Two cups of water (bubbled and cooled)
One tbsp. of scouring liquor

Method:

1. Take a clean glass bowl to make a mixture of scouring liquor, basic balsam of Perú oil, and tea tree oil. Stir well to mix them.
2. Combine aloe vera gel in the bowl and blend the mixture thoroughly.
3. Add bubbled and cooled water to the mixture and make a homogeneous mixture.
4. Sterilize a squirt bottle and pour the prepared balsam of Perú sanitizer in it using a channel.
5. Store the sanitizer bottle in a cool place and keep away from the direct sunlight.
6. It is essential to shake the sanitizer bottle when you use it.

Note: Balsam of Perú oil acts as an antifungal and antibacterial agent as per its properties.

Basil Sanitizer

Ingredients:

One tbsp. of scouring liquor
Two cups of water (bubbled and cooled)
Five drops of basil oil (basic)
Half tbsp. of aloe vera gel
Five drops of tea tree oil

Method:

1. Use a glass bowl to make a mixture of scouring liquor, tea tree oil, and basic basil oil. Stir well to combine them.
2. Then, combine aloe vera gel in the bowl and blend it into the mixture.
3. Mix water in the mixture and stir thoroughly to combine all the ingredients.
4. Sterilize a squirt bottle and pour the prepared basil sanitizer in it through a channel from the bowl.
5. Place the sanitizer bottle is a cool place to keep away from the direct sunlight.
6. You must shake the sanitizer bottle thoroughly before using it.

Note: Basil oil acts as an antibacterial agent according to its properties.

Bergamot Sanitizer

Ingredients:

One tbsp. of scouring liquor
Five drops of bergamot oil (basic)
Two cups of water (bubbled and cooled)
Five drops of tea tree oil
Half-tbsp. of aloe vera gel

Method:

1. Use a clean glass bowl for mixing scouring liquor, tea tree oil, and basic bergamot oil and stir them to combine well.
2. Then, mix aloe vera gel in the bowl and blend it thoroughly in the mixture.
3. Combine bubbled and cooled water in the mixture and stir it to mix all the ingredients completely.
4. Transfer the prepared bergamot sanitizer to a sterile dispenser through a pipe from the glass bowl.
5. Store the sanitizer dispenser in a cool place to protect from the heat of direct sunlight.
6. Don't forget to shake the sanitizer dispenser when you use it.

Note: Bergamot oil acts as an antibacterial agent as per its properties.

Black Pepper Oil Sanitizer

Ingredients:

One tbsp. of scouring liquor
Two cups of water (bubbled and cooled)
Five drops of tea tree oil
Half a tbsp. of aloe vera gel
Five drops of black pepper oil (basic)

Method:

1. Take a clean glass bowl and use it for mixing tea tree oil, basic black pepper oil, and scouring liquor. Stir them to mix well.
2. Then, combine aloe vera gel in the bowl and blend properly with the mixture.
3. Make a homogeneous mixture after mixing bubbled and cooled water in the bowl.
4. Sterilize squirt bottles and transfer the prepared black peeper oil sanitizer to them from the bowl through a channel.
5. Place the squirt bottles with sanitizer in a cool place to protect from the heat of direct sunlight.
6. Use the sanitizer after shaking the bottle thoroughly.

Citronella Sanitizer

Ingredients:

Half a tbsp. of aloe vera gel
Five drops of citronella oil (basic)
One tbsp. of scouring liquor
Two cups of water (bubbled and cooled)
Five drops of tea tree oil

Method:

1. Combine scouring liquor, tea tree oil, and basic citronella oil in a sterile glass bowl. Stir them to mix completely.
2. Include aloe vera gel in the bowl with the mixture and blend it properly.
3. Pour bubbled and cooled water into the bowl and stir the mixture to combine well.
4. Use sterile spray bottles to pour the prepared citronella sanitizer from the bowl with the help of a channel.
5. Store the sanitizer bottles is a cool place and maintain protection from the sunlight directly.
6. Shake well the sanitizer bottle when you use it.

Cidron Oil Sanitizer

Ingredients

Half a tbsp. of aloe vera gel
Five drops of tea tree oil
Two cups of water (bubbled and cooled)
One tbsp. if scouring liquor
Five drops of cidron oil (fundamental)

Method:

1. Use a clean glass bowl to make a mixture of fundamental cidron oil, scouring liquor, and tea tree oil. Stir it to combine well.
2. Then, blend the mixture thoroughly after mixing aloe vera gel in the bowl.
3. Add bubbled and cooled water to the bowl and prepare a homogeneous mixture.
4. Sterilize dispensers and empty the bowl by pouring the prepared cidron oil sanitizer into them using a channel.
5. Protect the sanitizer dispensers from the direct sunlight and store them in a cool place.
6. Don't forget to shake well the sanitizer dispenser before using it.

Salvia Sclarea Oil Sanitizer

Ingredients:

One tbsp. of scouring liquor
Five drops of salvia sclarea oil (fundamental)
Two cups of water (bubbled and cooled)
Five drops of tea tree oil
Half a tbsp. of aloe vera gel

Method:

1. Mix tea tree oil, scouring liquor, and fundamental salvia sclarea oil in a clean glass bowl. Stir them to combine well.
2. Blend the mixture thoroughly after adding the aloe vera gel in the bowl.
3. Again, blend well the mixture after pouring bubbled and cooled water in the glass bowl.
4. Use sterile spray bottles to store the prepared salvia sclarea sanitizer in them.
5. Place the sanitizer bottles in a cool place and protect them from the heat of the daylight.
6. Shake thoroughly the bottle when you use the sanitizer.

Melissa Oil Sanitizer

Ingredients:

One tbsp. of scouring liquor
Five drops of Melissa oil (basic)
Two cups of water (bubbled and cooled)
Five drops of tea tree oil
Half a tbsp. of aloe vera gel

Method:

1. Make a mixture of scouring liquor, tea tree oil, and basic Melissa oil in a sterile glass bowl. Stir them to mix well.
2. Combine aloe vera gel in the glass bowl and blend it completely in the mixture.
3. Add bubbled and cooled water in the bowl and stir well to prepare a homogeneous mixture.
4. Sterilize squirt bottles to transfer prepared sanitizer from the bowl through a channel.
5. Store the squirt bottles with sanitizer in a cool place and protect them from the sunlight directly.
6. It is essential to shake the bottle thoroughly when you use sanitizer.

Moringa Sanitizer

Ingredients:

One tbsp. of scouring liquor
Five drops of moringa oil (basic)
Two cups of water (bubbled and cooled)
Five drops of tea tree oil
Half a tbsp. of aloe vera gel

Method:

1. Use a clean glass bowl to combine scouring liquor, tea tree oil, and basic moringa oil and stir well the mixture.
2. Bled the mixture thoroughly after adding aloe vera gel to the bowl.
3. Make the right consistency of the mixture after pouring the bubbled and cooled water in the bowl.
4. Fill the sterile spray bottles with prepared moringa sanitizer through a channel.
5. Place the spray bottles with sanitizer in a cool place to protect them from daylight directly.
6. Use the sanitizer after shaking it thoroughly.

Thyme Oil and Vitamin E Sanitizer

Ingredients:

One tsp. of vitamin E oil
Two drops of tea tree oil (basic)
Three tbsps. of aloe vera gel
Three drops of thyme oil (basic)
One tbsp. of witch hazel

Method:

1. Sterilize a glass bowl and combine witch hazel, basic thyme oil, vitamin E oil, and tea tree oil in it. Stir well to mix completely.
2. Blend the mixture thoroughly after adding aloe vera gel in the bowl.
3. Use sterile spray bottles to store prepared sanitizer. Also, use a channel to transfer the prepared sanitizer from the bowl to the spray bottles.
4. Place the spray bottles with sanitizer in a cool place to protect them from the direct daylight.
5. Use the sanitizer after shaking the bottle thoroughly.

Rose Mary and Lemongrass Sanitizer

Ingredients:

Twenty drops of tea tree oil
Two tbsps. of water (bubbled and cooled)
Five drops of lemongrass oil (basic)
Two tbsps. of witch hazel
Five drops of rosemary oil (basic)
One tbsp. of glycerin (vegetable)

Method:

1. Use a sterile glass container to mix witch hazel, basic rosemary oil, tea tree oil, and basic lemongrass oil and stir well to mix them.
2. Blend the mixture completely after adding vegetable glycerin in the bowl.
3. Then, combine bubbled and cooled water in the bowl and make a homogeneous mixture.
4. Use a channel to pour prepared sanitizer into sterile dispensers from the bowl.
5. Keep the sanitizer dispensers in a cool place to protect them from the sunlight directly.
6. Shake well the dispenser when you use it.

Thieves Oil and Vitamin E Oil Sanitizer

Ingredients:

A one-third cup of witch hazel (liquor-free)
A one-fourth tsp. of vitamin E oil
A two-third cup of aloe vera gel (pure)
Fifteen drops of criminal oil mix (basic)

Method:

1. Make a mixture of vitamin E oil, witch hazel, and basic criminal oil mix in a clean glass bowl and stir well.
2. Blend the mixture thoroughly after mixing aloe vera gel in the bowl and make a homogeneous mixture.
3. Sterilize squirt bottles and transfer the prepared sanitizer from the bowl to the squirt bottles using a channel.
4. Maintain protection for the bottles with sanitizer from the heat of the direct sunlight and place them in a cool place.
5. Don't forget to shake well the sanitizer bottles before using it.

Aloe Vera-Free Sanitizer

Ingredients:

Two drops of vitamin E oil
Five drops of orange oil (fundamental)
Sterile water (as per need)
Five drops of lemon oil (fundamental)
Five drops of tea tree oil
Two tbsps. of vodka

Method:

1. Use a clean glass bowl to mix vodka, vitamin E oil, and fundamental oils of lemon, orange, and tea tree oil. Stir the mixture to mix them well.
2. Take small-sized spray bottles to fill sterile water nearly the whole bottle.
3. Transfer the prepared sanitizer from the glass bowl to the spray bottles using a channel.
4. Place the spray bottles with sanitizer in a cool place to protect them from the direct sunlight.
5. Don't forget to shake the sanitizer bottle thoroughly before using it.

Rosemary and Aloe Vera Sanitizer

Ingredients:

A one-quarter cup of vodka
One tbsp. of lavender slave (natural)
Half-cup of aloe vera (juice)
Ten to twenty drops of rosemary oil (basic)

Method:

1. Use a clean glass bowl to mix aloe vera juice, rosemary oil, natural lavender oil, and vodka. Stir well to combine all the ingredients with each other.
2. Pour the prepared sanitizer in sterile dispensers from the glass bowl through a channel.
3. Store the dispensers with sanitizer in a cool place and protect them from the heat of the direct sunlight.
4. It is essential to shake the dispenser thoroughly when you use the sanitizer.

Almond Oil Sanitizer

Ingredients:

A one-quarter tsp. of almond oil
One cup of aloe vera gel
Thirty drops of tea tree oil (basic)
One tbsp. of witch hazel (concentrate)
Ten drops of lavender oil (basic)

Method:

1. Make a mixture of concentrated witch hazel, almond oil, basic lavender oil, and tea tree oil in a clean glass bowl.
2. Combine aloe vera gel in the bowl and blend the mixture thoroughly to make a homogeneous mixture.
3. Pour the prepared sanitizer in sterile spray bottles from the bowl through a channel.
4. Keep the sanitizer bottles in a cool place to protect them from the direct sunlight.
5. It is important to shake well the bottles before using the sanitizer.

Alcohol-Free Witch Hazel Sanitizer

Ingredients:

One tbsp. of witch hazel (alcohol-free)
A one-quarter tsp. of vitamin E oil
One tbsp. of aloe vera gel
Thirty drops of tea tree oil

Method:

1. Take a sterile glass bowl to make a mixture of alcohol-free witch hazel, tea tree oil, and vitamin E oil and stir it to combine well.
2. Combine aloe vera gel in the bowl and blend the mixture thoroughly to mix all the ingredients with each other.
3. Pour the prepared sanitizer in the sterile dispensers from the bowl through a channel.
4. Keep the dispensers with sanitizer in a cool place to resist the heat of the direct sunlight.
5. You must shake well the dispenser before using the sanitizer.

White Vinegar Sanitizer

Ingredients:

Half-cup of refined water
A one-quarter cup of refined white vinegar

Method:

1. Use a clean glass bowl to mix refined white vinegar with water and stir well to make a homogeneous solution.
2. Sterilize spray bottles and pour the prepared sanitizer into them from the glass bowl using a pipe.
3. Keep the sanitizer bottles in a cool place and resist the direct sunlight from them.
4. Don't forget to shake the bottle completely when you use the sanitizer.

Apple Cider Vinegar Sanitizer

Ingredients:

Half-cup of aloe vera gel
A one-quarter cup of vinegar (apple juice)

Method:

1. Mix aloe vera gel with apple juice vinegar in a clean glass bowl. Blend them until they mix completely to each other.
2. Sterilize dispensers and transfer the prepared sanitizer in the dispensers through a channel.
3. Place the sanitizer dispensers in a cool place to resist the heat of the daylight directly.
4. Always shake the dispenser thoroughly before using the sanitizer.

Orange and Cinnamon Sanitizer

Ingredients:

Ten drops of cinnamon oil (fundamental)
A One-quarter cup of aloe vera gel
Twenty drops of orange oil (fundamental)
Five drops of rosemary oil (fundamental)
Ten drops of lavender oil (fundamental)
Five drops of clove oil (fundamental)

Method:

1. Combine the fundamental oils of clove, orange, lavender, cinnamon, and rosemary in a clean glass bowl and stir well to combine them well.
2. Blend the mixture thoroughly after adding the aloe vera gel to the bowl and make a homogeneous mixture.
3. Use a pipe to transfer the prepared sanitizer to the sterile squirt bottles from the bowl.
4. Maintain essential protection from the direct sunlight by placing the squirt bottles with sanitizer in a cool place.
5. Always shake the bottle completely when you use the sanitizer.

Melaleuca and white Fir Sanitizer

Ingredients:

Fifteen drops of white fir oil (fundamental)
Half-tsp. of vitamin E oil
Twenty drops of melaleuca oil (fundamental)
Half-cup of aloe vera gel (unadulterated)
Fifteen drops of lemon oil (fundamental)
A one-quarter cup each of
- Water (refined)
- Witch hazel (liquor-free)

Method:

1. Make a mixture of fundamental oil of white fir, lemon, and melaleuca, vitamin E oil, and liquor-free witch hazel in a clean glass bowl and stir them to combine well.
2. Mix unadulterated aloe vera gel in the bowl and blend the mixture thoroughly.
3. Then, pour refined water in the bowl and blend the mixture again to make a homogeneous mixture.
4. Transfer the prepared sanitizer to clean dispensers from the bowl using a channel.
5. Store the sanitizer dispensers in a cool place to protect them from direct sunlight.
6. Don't forget to shake the dispenser thoroughly before using the sanitizer.

Tea Tree Oil and Castile Soap Sanitizer

Ingredients:

One tsp. of Castile cleanser
Ten drops of tea tree oil (basic)
Six ounces of water (bubbled and cooled)

Method:

1. Take a sterile glass bowl and mix basic tea tree oil with Castile cleanser. Stir them to combine well.
2. Then, add bubbled and cooled water to the bowl and prepare a homogeneous mixture after blending them thoroughly.
3. Empty the bowl by pouring the prepared sanitizer into clean spray bottles through a channel.
4. Place the spray bottles containing sanitizer in a cool place and protect them from the daylight directly.
5. You must sake the bottle thoroughly before the use of sanitizer.

Coconut Oil Sanitizer

Ingredients:

Twenty drops of cheat youthful living oil
Two tsps. coconut oil
Half a tsp. of ocean salt
Distilled water (as per need)

Method:

1. Take ocean salt in a sterile and glass made spray bottle.
2. Leave the bottle for 5 minutes in a safe place after adding cheat youthful living oil to the ocean salt.
3. Now, fill the larger part of the bottle with distilled water.
4. Then, combine coconut oil in the bottle.
5. Shake the spray bottle with the mixture thoroughly to ensure the mixing of all the ingredients to each other.
6. Store the sanitizer bottle in a cool place and keep safe from the direct sunlight.
7. Use the sanitizer after shaking the bottle thoroughly.

Frankincense and Lavender Oil Sanitizer

Ingredients:

One tbsp. of aloe vera gel
Twenty bring down doTERRAon Defenses oil (basic)
Boiled and cooled water (as per need)

Method:

1. Mix the basic oil and aloe vera gel in a sterile spray bottle.
2. Then, fill the remaining part of the bottle with boiled and cooled water.
3. Shake well spray bottle to ensure the mixing completely.
4. Store the sanitizer bottle in a cool place to keep safe from the heat of the direct daylight.
5. It is essential to shake the sanitizer bottle thoroughly before using it.

Virus Shield Sanitizer

Ingredients:

Six drops of lavender oil (fundamental)
Two drops of water (refined)
Two tbsps. of isopropyl liquor (90%)
Half a tsp. of vitamin E oil
Three tbsps. of aloe vera gel
Ten drops of tea tree oil

Method:

1. Take a clean glass bowl to mix vitamin E oil, fundamental lavender oil, and tea tree oil. Stir them with a clean spoon or wooden spatula to blend well.
2. Then, combine isopropyl liquor and aloe vera gel in the bowl and blend the mixture thoroughly.
3. Make the perfect consistency of the sanitizer by adding two drops of refined water.
4. Fill a clean dispenser with the prepared sanitizer from the bowl.
5. Place the dispenser filled with prepared sanitizer in a cool place to keep safe from the heat of the direct daylight.
6. Always use the sanitizer after shaking the dispenser well.

Floral Sanitizer

Ingredients:

A one-quarter tsp. of vitamin E oil
A two-third cup of isopropyl liquor (91%)
Ten drops of almond oil
A one-third cup of aloe vera gel
Ten drops of rose oil

Method:

1. Combine rose oil and almond oil in a clean glass bowl and stir them with a wooden spatula to mix well.
2. Then, blend the mixture thoroughly after mixing aloe vera gel and isopropyl liquor in the bowl.
3. Include vitamin E oil in the glass bowl and make a homogeneous mixture by blending completely all the ingredients within the mixture of the bowl.
4. Use a channel to pour the prepared sanitizer in a sterile spray bottle from the bowl.
5. Store the spray bottle containing sanitizer in a cool place to keep safe from the sunlight directly.
6. It is important to shake the bottle adequately before using the sanitizer.

Citrus Blend Sanitizer

Ingredients:

Three drops each of
- Orange oil (fundamental)
- Ylang oil (fundamental
- Lavender oil (fundamental)

Half-cup of aloe vera gel (unadulterated)
A one-quarter tbsp. of vitamin E oil
A two-third cup of witch hazel (concentrate)

Method:

1. Make a mixture of fundamental lavender oil, orange oil, Yland oil, and vitamin E oil in a clean glass bowl. Stir them using a wooden spatula to combine well.
2. Mix witch hazel and aloe vera gel in the glass bowl and blend the mixture completely to combine well.
3. Fill a spray bottle with prepared sanitizer using a channel form the bowl.
4. Store the sanitizer bottle in a cool place to keep safe from the heat of the sunlight directly.
5. Don't forget to shake the sanitizer bottle before using it.

Extra Citrus Hand Sanitizer

Ingredients:

Three drops each of
- Wild orange oil (fundamental)
- Lemongrass oil (fundamental)
- Bergamot oil (fundamental)

Two tbsps. of aloe vera gel
One tbsp. of scouring liquor

Method:

1. Use a sterile glass bowl to mix fundamental oil of lemongrass, wild orange, bergamot, scouring liquor, and aloe vera gel. Blend the mixture thoroughly to mix all the ingredients.
2. Fill a sterile squirt bottle with prepared sanitizer using a channel from the glass bowl.
3. Place the sanitizer bottle in a cool place to protect it from the direct daylight.
4. Always shake the bottle well when you use the sanitizer.

Vanilla and Lavender Sanitizer

Ingredients:

Ten drops of vanilla oil (fundamental)
A two-third cup of isopropyl alcohol
Five drops of lavender oil (fundamental)
A one-third cup of aloe vera gel

Method:

1. Combine fundamental oil of lavender and vanilla in a sterile glass bowl and stir well to mix them.
2. Then, blend well the mixture after adding isopropyl alcohol and aloe vera gel in the glass bowl.
3. Transfer the prepared sanitizer in a sterile spray bottle form the bowl using a channel.
4. Store the sanitizer bottle in a cool place and protect from direct sunlight.
5. Don't forget to shake the bottle well to get the right consistency before using the sanitizer.

Fresh Mint Sanitizer

Ingredients:

Three drops each of
- Eucalyptus oil (fundamental)
- Peppermint oil (fundamental)

Half-cup of aloe vera gel (unadulterated)
Two drops of coconut oil
A two-third cup of witch hazel (concentrate)

Method:

1. Take a clean glass bowl and make a mixture of fundamental oil of peppermint and eucalyptus with coconut oil in the glass bowl. Stir well to mix them.
2. Then, combine concentrate witch hazel and aloe vera gel in the bowl and blend well the mixture to make a homogeneous mixture.
3. Fill a clean dispenser with prepared sanitizer from the bowl through a channel.
4. Store the dispenser with sanitizer in a cool place to keep safe from direct sunlight.
5. You should shake the dispenser appropriately before using the sanitizer.

Spicy Sanitizer

Ingredients:

Ten drops each of
- Sage oil (fundamental)
- Thyme oil (fundamental)

A two-third cup of witch hazel
Five drops of jojoba oil (bearer oil)
A one-third cup of aloe vera gel

Method:

1. Mix fundamental oil of thyme, sage, and jojoba oil in a sterile glass bowl and stir the for mixing well.
2. Then, blend completely the mixture after adding witch hazel and aloe vera gel to the glass bowl.
3. Pour the prepared sanitizer with accurate consistency in a sterile squirt bottle from the bowl using a channel.
4. Place the squirt bottle containing sanitizer in a cool place and protect it from the heat of the sunlight directly.
5. Shake the bottle thoroughly before using the sanitizer.

Tropical Sanitizer

Ingredients:

Ten drops of orange oil
A two-third cup of isopropyl alcohol (90%)
Ten tsps. of coconut oil
A one-third cup of aloe vera gel

Method:

1. Use a clean glass bowl to combine coconut oil with orange oil and stir well to mix them.
2. Then, add isopropyl alcohol and aloe vera gel to the bowl and blend them completely to make a homogenous mixture.
3. Transfer the prepared sanitizer with proper consistency in a sterile spray bottle using a channel from the glass bowl.
4. Protect the sanitizer bottle from direct sunlight by placing it in a cool place.
5. Don't forget to shake the bottle appropriately when you are going to use the sanitizer.

Conclusion

Thank you for making it through to the end of *Make Your Own Hand Sanitizer: A Step-By-Step Guide To Make Your Own Natural Homemade Hand Wipes, Spray, Sanitizer, and Liquid Soap to Kill Germs, Viruses and Bacteria For a Healthier Lifestyle*, let's hope it was informative and able to provide you with all of the tools you need to achieve your goals whatever they may be.

With the COVID-19 virus spreading like wildfire, hygiene has become more important than ever before. Every doctor and health professional is advising people to use hand sanitizers and to wash your hands after every few minutes. You should also carry a sanitizer with you whenever you are traveling somewhere, even if it means going to the local market, especially amidst this global crisis.

If someone has already encountered some disease or flu and if you have come in contact with that person, then you will have to wash your hands before you use them for any purpose whatsoever. What is every scarier is that you cannot see the virus or bacteria around you and so you do not know whether an object is contaminated or not. That is why it is best that you sanitizer your hands from time to time. And now that you have completed the book, I am sure you have plenty of variations at your hand so that you do not have to stick to one sanitizer for a long time. So, go to the supermarket and get all the things you need and make your own sanitizer at home.

If you're interested read also **Homemade Face Masks**

The Complete Guide To Learn How To Make Your Protective Masks at Home With Step-by-Step Descriptions and Graphic Representations by the same author!

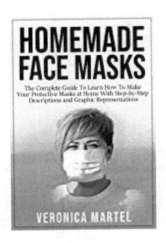

Finally, if you found this book useful in any way, a review on Amazon is always appreciated!

CPSIA information can be obtained
at www.ICGtesting.com
Printed in the USA
LVHW050048091220
673659LV00034B/908